COW KEEPING IN INDIA

A Simple and Practical Book on their Care and Treatment, their various Breeds, and the Means of rendering them Profitable

Fifth Edition

S.N. SINHA, *G.B.V.C., B.V.S.*
Professor of Surgery and Obstetrics,
Bengal Veterinary College, Belgachia

BIOTECH

2023

Biotech Books

ISBN 978-81-7622-098-9

Published by : **BIOTECH BOOKS**
4762-63/23, Ansari Road, Darya Ganj,
New Delhi - 110002
Phones : 011 4300 3222
Email : biotechbooks@yahoo.co.in

PRINTED IN INDIA

Foreword to Fifth Edition

I have just perused, "Revised Fifth Edition of Cow keeping in India," prior to publication by Messrs Thacker, Spink & Company, Limited, Kolkata.

The revisions and additions cover a large field of recent discovery, both in the theory and practice of Cattle-breeding and Cow keeping in India, the original text also being enhanced by many clear and instructive illustrations.

I cannot imagine any household, desirous of getting the best out of life in the shape of good healthy milk, being without such an encyclopaedia of the cow; and even to the expert dairyman much of new interest and instruction can be found in these pages. It is a most pleasurable and readable book and at the same time as accurate as any text book.

The editor (Mr. S. N. Sinha) lays much to his credit in the elaborate and accurate revision he has made of this well-founded and popular book.

A.D. MacGregor
F.R.C.V.S, F.Z.S., I.V.S.
Principal, Bengal Veterinary College
Kolkata

Preface to Fifth Edition

For the production of the Fifth Edition of this work I have been entrusted by the publishers with, I believe, no mean task for one man to accomplish. I have, however, endeavoured as best as I could to put as much practical and theoretical information within easy reach of the reader as is consistent with the times. A revision, in all conscience, entails not only changes here and there in the existing text but also the judicious omission of old or obsolete material, and the supplementing of necessary and useful information by bringing it into line with present-day practice. In producing the present edition, therefore, I have been only too glad to avail myself of the kind inspiration and help of my Principal–Mr. A.D. MacGregor of the Bengal Veterinary College–and of Mr. R.T. Davis, Principal of the Bihar and Orissa Veterinary College, without whom the task would have been more arduous: to them I take this opportunity of expressing my deep gratitude. Mr. MacGregor has also been kind enough to write a "Foreword" to the edition unsolicited. I am also deeply indebted to my friend and colleague Mr. K.K. Banerjee for suggesting some additions and corrections.

As it has been found from experience that indigenous medicines answer well in the diseases of indigenous animals and that these are cheap and easily procurable, I have given some recipes with vernacular equivalents which may satisfy Indian requirements. This is a new feature in this addition, another being that a few pages have been added giving the names of certain very common place indigenous drugs, their Bengali, Hindi and English names, their application in particular diseases and dosage.

In conclusion, I venture to hope that this edition may prove helpful to cow-keepers, students and practical dairymen and that it may assist them in the proper care, management and treatment of the cattle under their charge.

S.N. Sinha
Bengal Veterinary College
Kolkata

Preface to First Edition

When I commenced keeping cows I often wished for a simple and practical book on cattle and their care and treatment in India, and I have frequently heard the same wish expressed by others. If I had such a Part 1 would have been saved a great deal of needless worry and loss.

There are many books on cattle and their care in Europe; but though these books are a great help to people in Europe, they are of no practical use to us in India. The climate and soil of India are different from those of England and other European countries, and the cattle here need different treatment. Some books have been published on Indian cattle, but the best of these is far from being complete.

I have for the past eighteen years kept my own cows; and for many years have myself undertaken their medical treatment. I have also carefully read all the books. I could procure on cattle of all descriptions, both English and Indian.

The knowledge I have thus acquired may be of some service to others, so I herein give my experience for what it may be worth.

The method of treatment that I herein recommend for cows in health and sickness, is what I have most successfully adopted for many years. I generally adhere to homeopathy, and in most cases it is the only effectual method of treatment; but in many cases I have found the Indian remedies very effcacious. I do not hesitate to prescribe the most effective remedy, be it homeopathic or Indian medicine, or anything else.

As I have said, I have carefully read many books on cattle, their diseases and treatment; and in my notes I have tried, as much as possible, to avoid even the appearance of plagiarism. But it is impossible for any two persons writing on one subject, and especially a subject like this, to avoid often saying the same thing, and sometimes saying it in the same words.

Amongst the first things I earned when I commenced life were: 1st, if I wished to succeed in anything, I must do the work myself and not trust another person to do it for me; 2nd, I must attend to every detail with equal fidelity. As with other matters in life, so with the keeping of cows-personal care and supervision, and the strictest attention to details, are absolutely essential to success. The least negligence or delay will cause much loss and disappointment. If a person has not the inclination or time to look after his pets and live-stock, he should not attempt to keep any.

The busiest people need regular recreation from their regular work. Without it, it is impossible to maintain good health or mental equilibrium. The greatest minds have experienced this, and it is hazardous to ignore this rule of health. Some persons choose gardening or carpentry as a recreation, others, again, riding or some game of sport. But keeping cows is a very healthful and, at the same time, profitable pastime.

I have often thought, if more European and well-to-do Indian families in this country were to keep cows there would be less disease, and less annoyance about procuring pure milk, butter and ghee, and there would also be a great improvement in the breed of cattle. Keeping cows does not take much time or money, if one knows how to do it properly. But this knowledge is not acquired without careful study and some experience.

I am convinced that very few persons in India know how to properly care for cattle when in health, or treat them when sick. Most people trust the care of their cattle entirely to their servants. I have seen many splendid cows utterly spoiled, and a number die from sheer neglect or mismanagement.

There are a number of good Veterinary Surgeons and other gentlemen practising medicine in every town, and it would be more economical in the end to consult the best of them than to trust the stupid servants.

ISA Tweed

Contents

Foreword to Fifth Edition iii
Preface to Fifth Edition v
Preface to First Edition vii

Part 1

1. **The Advantages of Keeping Cows** 3

   Pure milk; Cheapness; Calf; Other produce; Keeping cows is a pleasure and a saving

2. **Breeds of Cattle** 6

   Montgomery; Sind; Hansi or Hissar; Nagauri; Nellore or Ongole; Gir; Kankreji; Goorgaira; Mooltan and Amritsar; Krishna Valley; Kangayam; Mysore; Dhanni; Awankari; Bengal; Bihar; Bhagalpore; Darjeeling; Patna; English and Australian; Cross-bred English; The breed to get

3. **Buying Cows** 51

   Quantity of milk required; Servants' tricks; Buying a cow with a calf; Buying a cow in calf; Selecting a cow that has calved the first time; To judge a young cow; General appearance; Pay good price

4. **Points in a Good Cow** 57

   Outward appearance; Temper; Colour; Quality of milk; Blind nipples; The cow's udder; A big bag; The shape; Distending udder; The teats; Scarred cows; Age; Number of calves a cow has had; A good milker; A slinker; Calves; The wedge shape

5. **Food**

Proper care and treatment of milking cows; Food; Kinds of grain; Bran; Sharps and middlings; Quantity of food; Effects of the different kinds of food; Preparation of food; Cost of food; Green food; Doob; Jowar; Sorghum poisoning; Straw; Hay; Bhoosa; Salt; Drink; Silage

6. **House and Utensils** 75

The Cow-house; Space; Keeping the floor clean and dry; Drains; Utensils; Cistern; Mode of tying; The yard; Other houses

7. **Attendants** 82

The Servants' disposition of mind; Fidelity

8. **Washing, Grooming and Exercise** 84

Washing; Grooming; Exercise; Protection

9. **Breeding** 86

Breeding; It is cheaper to breed one's own cows; The art of breeding; The dual purpose cow for India

10. **Bulls** 93

The necessity for a bull; Indian bulls v. English bulls; Points in a good Indian bull; Age; Care and attention; Food; Utensils; House and grooming; Fat; Keeping him separate; Serving; Over-starving; The sire

11. **Bullocks** 98

Bullocks and buffaloes; Points in a good bullock; Food; Grooming and cleaning; Water; Rearing

12. **Dry Cows** 100

Selling dry cows; Keeping dry cows; Advantage; Food; Over-feeding; The reason why; Exercise; Care; Protection from disease; Cleanliness; Time of pregnancy; Selling dry cows to butchers; How to dispose of dry cows and young calves

13. **Management of Cows When Calving** 106

Signs of the time; Labour approaching; Progress of labour; Assistance needed; Treatment after birth; Drink and food; Illness; Falling of womb; Milking

14. Calves: Their Value, Management and House 111

Value of calves; Food and care; Tying; House; Shelter; Ticks and lice; Older calves; Careful treatment; Treat the cows kindly; Why so many calves die

15. Points in a Good Calf 117

Good bull-calf; Good cow-calf

16. Castrating Calves 118

Castrating when young; Mode; Effect; Great care; Proper time; Evils of late castration

17. Taking the Bull 120

Very important matter; Early months of pregnancy; Signs; When a cow comes into season; Symptoms; The time a cow remain in season; Troublesome cows; Barren cows; A good bull; Putting the cow to the bull

18. Barren Cows 124

Cause of sterility; Remedy; Barrenness in dairy cattle

19. Age of Cattle and Names at Different Ages 128

Age; Name at different ages; Indian names

20. Price of Cattle 133

Prices of cows; Bulls; Bullocks; Calves

21. Milk 135

Quantity of milk; Quality of milk; Lactometer; Duration of milk; Papeeta; Art of milking; Young cows need careful milkers; Process of milking; Milking utensils; When the calf dies; Every drop of milk must be extracted; Cows holding up milk; Forcing supplies; Importance of regularity in milking

22. Cream 143

Watered milk; Cream; Keeping milk good; Skimmed milk; Boiling milk; Susceptibilty of milk

23. Butter 146

Boiled and unboiled milk; Collecting cream; Process of butter-making; The indigenous churn; Dazey churn; Cleanliness; Preserving butter; Sweet or sour cream

24. Ghee 151

Making ghee; Clarifying ghee

25. Curd, Cheese, and Tyer 153

Making curd; Cream cheese; Tyer

26. Lice, Ticks, Flies, etc. 155

27. The Seasons of the Year 157

Cold weather; Hot weather; Rains

28. Cattle-Dung 159

Cattle-dung; Profit; Manure-pit

29. Grazing Fields 160

Providing fodder; Amount of land needed; Fertility of land; The best time to manure; Preparation of land; Draining; Doob; Lucerne grass; Green food; Sorghum poison at different stages of growth

30. Dairy-Farming 165

Certain things necessary; India one of the best countries for dairy-farming; Experience; Capital; The position of the dairy-farm; The class of cattle needed; Dry cows; Breeding for the dairy; Bulls; Important matters; Profitable and unprofitable cows; Buffaloes; Some difficulties.

31. Breeding and Rearing Farms, Dry-Cow Farming and Cattle-Shows 177

Breeding farms; Rearing farms; Dry-cow farming; Cattle-shows

32. What Experts Say 185

Cattle-Breeding in India; What India needs; The basis upon which to work; How to obtain what is needed; Lines on which to work: Mendelian theory; The imported fixed line; Milch cattle in India; Breeding milch cattle; Standards of excellence in selection; Influence of the sire; Care and management; Food supply; Improvement a slow process; Methods employed; Grading; Cross-breeding; Developing the heifer; Rearing of calves in India; A useful calf meal; Rearing of calves on Government military farms; Artificial milk of calves and pigs; Improvement of cattle in Bengal

Part 2

1. **Diseases of Cattle, Goats and Sheep** 211

2. **Some Common Complaints** 216

   Cough; Weak eyes; Inflammation of the eyes; Mange; Broken horns; Leech in the nose; Wounds and bruises; Enlarged papillae; Wasting in calves; Cold or catarrh; Sprains; Dislocation; Sore feet; Costiveness; Irregular teeth; The navel ill; Sore teats

3. **Dangerous but not Contagious Diseases** 226

   Calving-After-pains-The after-birth-Flooding; Inflammation of the womb; Slipping down of the womb; Swollen udder-Cure for mastitis-Treatment for lumpy milk-Cause of ropy milk; Rheumatism; Paralysis, Hoven; Grain-sick; Fardel-bound; Choking; Red-water; Indigestion and diarrhoea; Epilepsy; Apoplexy; Inflammation of the brain; Colic; Parasitic warbles; Hydatids; Inflammation of the bowels; Hernia; Jaundice; Poisoning; Abscess

4. **Contagious and Fatal Diseases** 253

   Rinderpest; Foot-and-mouth disease; Malignant sore-throat; Bronchitis; Bronchitis from worms; Black-quarter; Dysentery; Slinking; Cow-pox; Milk fever; White scours in calves; Worms in the intestines; Tuberculosis; Anthrax; Rabies

Recipes 281

Recipes of Indigenous and Other Drugs for Diseases etc. 284

Breeder's Table 293

Weights and Measures 295

Indian Names of Some Cattle Diseases 298

Indigenous Drugs with Their Vernacular Names and Purposes 299

Index 303

Part 1

Chapter 1

The Advantages of Keeping Cows

Cows are kept by few for luxury, by some as a matter of business and by many for the sake of necessity. Cow keeping, if carried out properly, can be made paying and profitable.

Pure Milk

The first advantage derived from keeping one's own cows is, one gets pure and fresh milk. Pure and fresh milk is very essential to health; some persons do not drink milk, but they eat milk products, *e.g.*, cheese, dahi, butter, and ghee. If the milk be impure, the butter, ghee, etc., made from it must also be impure. Feeding children with adulterated, milk, butter, etc., brings in deficiency diseases, *e.g.*, Rickets, and acts as a poison to the consumer. Moreover, diseases like Cholera, Typhoid, Dysentery, etc., can also be conveyed to the human system through the agency of milk.

Too much stress cannot be put upon the necessity for having pure and fresh milk; but it is difficult to procure such an article from gowallas or ordinary people dealing in milk.

If people only knew what milk obtained from most of the gowallas contained, they would never again drink such stuff. Many gowallas are not at all scrupulous about the quality of water they put into the milk. Some of them dip their dirty clothes into stagnant filthy pools and wring the water out into the milk they are carrying to their customers. They have also been seen plunging their dirty hands in the milk. Many of them adulterate their milk with chalk and water, finely-sifted flour and water, yellow sugar, *batasha* and water, and innumerable other things that only the gowalla's ingenious mind could suggest. It is believed that in order to deceive the customer when using Lactometer some enterprising spirits among them dilute Swiss tinned-milk with water, and adulterate their milk with it. Some add water to buffalo's milk to bring it to the consistency of cow's milk and mix this with the latter. Buffalo's milk being very rich in butter fat (twice as much as cow's milk), a lot of water has to be added to it to make it as this as cow's milk. Mashed plantain is largely used for mixing with butter, as well as margarine.

These admixtures cannot but prove extremely injurious to the health of the consumer. It is exceedingly difficult for persons to guard against these dangers, especially when their servants are leagued together with the gowallas.

Cheapness

The second advantage gained by keeping cows is cheapness. The daily cost of feeding and keeping a cow should not ordinarily exceed three-fourths the price of the milk she gives. If she gives twelve pounds of milk per day, and the price of milk be two annas per pound, her food and keep should not ordinarily cost more than twelve annas per day. In some places fodder and grain are very dear, but milk is also proportionately dear in these places. For instance, in Kolkata the price of good milk is one rupee for four to six pounds; so if a cow gives only twelve pounds a day in Kolkata, it is not too much to spend Re.1 a day on her food and keep. A large cow, properly fed and giving from twenty to twenty-four pounds of milk, should never cost more than one rupee and annas eight a day for her food and keep even in Kolkata.

It is always more profitable to keep a cow giving a large quantity of milk than one that gives only a small quantity. A good cow will give from sixteen to twenty-four pounds or more a day when in full milk, and the cost of her keep and food will not exceed from a fourth to half the value of her milk. The surplus milk can be sold or made into butter and ghee for home use or for sale. Milk, butter and ghee will always find a ready sale; thus there need not be the least waste.

Calf

Besides the profit from the milk, there is the calf. If the calf be of a good breed, and proportionately developed, at ten months of age it will sell for from fifteen to thirty rupees.

Other Produce

Then, again there is the dung. Some people make a great deal of profit from this article. The dung-should be gathered every day, and preserved for either manure or fuel. It should be made into cakes or rolls, and dried and sold as fuel, or else a pit should be dug, and the dung and urine collected into it every day. Cow-dung and urine make splendid manure, The dung of one cow should fetch from eight annas to one rupee a month.

There is money even in the hide, horns, and bones of the cow when she dies.

Keeping Cows is a Pleasure and a Saving

By having one's own cows good milk and butter can be had and for less than one would have to pay for inferior milk and butter bought from the gowalla. But if the cow be left solely to the care and mercy of servants, she will soon become a troublesome and expensive thing; whereas the wicked servants will reap the profit from her.

The wife of a military officer, who has lived many years in India, writes: "A twenty years' experience, during which I have kept a record of every cow bought and sold and every calf born, enables me to assert that cows properly looked after are an economy. A cow purchased is, if well managed, so much capital; a calf born is so much increase on your capital, and the cost of mother's feed and keep is more than balanced by the milk and butter she supplies. I have kept cows in the hills and in the plains, and I have also been without cows, and my account books show that I have paid more for milk and butter when I bought them than I expended in the food and keep of my cows when I had them, and that in the latter case there was always plenty of dairy produce and to spare; whereas when I had to purchase, milk and butter had to be obtained sparingly and expended carefully. This is a great consideration in a large family, where, for the sake of the young people, milk and butter should be generously given out."-*Cows in India*.

Chapter 2

Breeds of Cattle

There are several distinct breeds of cattle in India. To ensure success in the dairy and farm, it is of the utmost importance that the best milking breeds be selected.

Some people are penny-wise and pound-foolish, and will buy cows of no stable breed whatever, and of very inferior milking qualities, rather than pay a decent price for a good and pedigreed one. An ordinary cow can be bought for a few rupees, but she will give little or no milk, and her feed and keep will cost more than her milk is worth. Besides, her calf will sell for hardly anything. This is a great loss. It is always more profitable to keep a good cow that will give the required amount of milk than to keep three or four inferior ones that will in the aggregate give that quantity. Four inferior cows will cost more to feed and keep than one or two good ones will. And the one or two good-ones can be given better care and attention than it is possible to give the three o four inferior ones; and without proper care and attention no cow will give her full milk.

Best Breeds of Cattle in India

Montgomery

Locally known as the Sahniwal or Teli breed. The cows are usually from 48 to 50 inches high, and the bulls from 52 to 58 inches. The head is long; forehead rather narrow; fairly short horns; rather large, hanging ears; short and thick neck; fair-size hump; the back is slightly curved and the back long and rises generally an inch or so at the croup; tail long and rather thin; the legs are fine and strong; feet large; the skin is thin and the coat fine; the dewlap is large; the sheath in the male, and the fold of skin under the abdomen in the

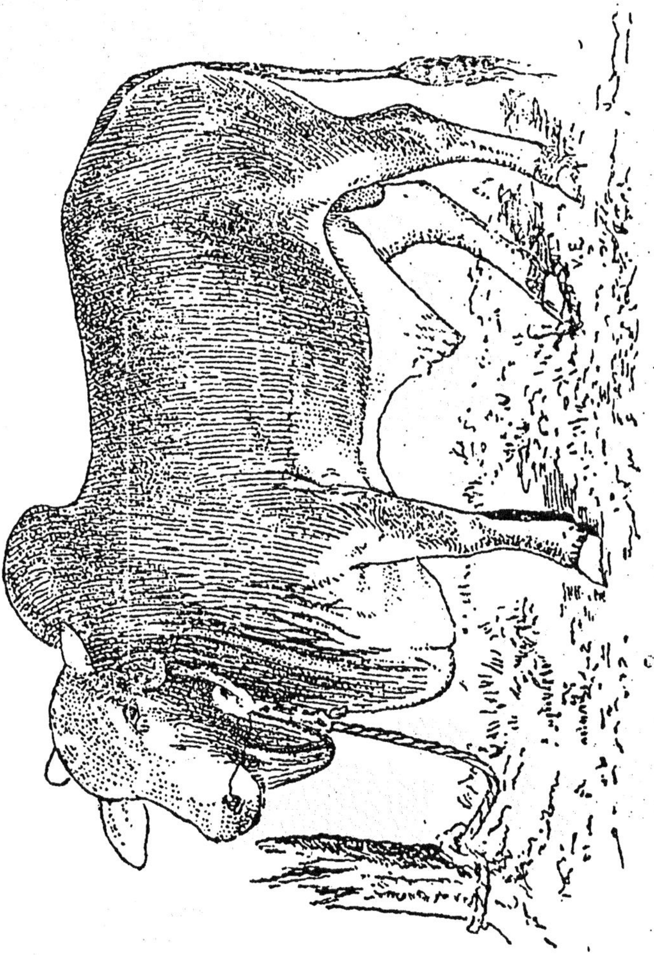

Fig. 1: Montgomery Bull

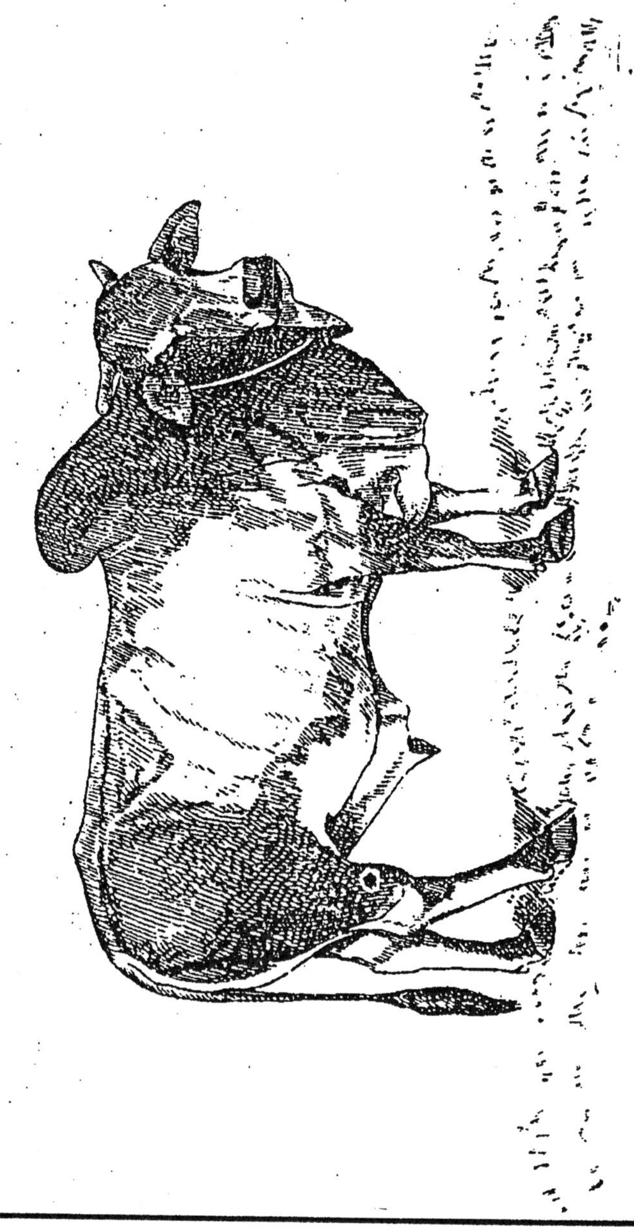

Fig. 2: Montgomery Bull (Amritsari)

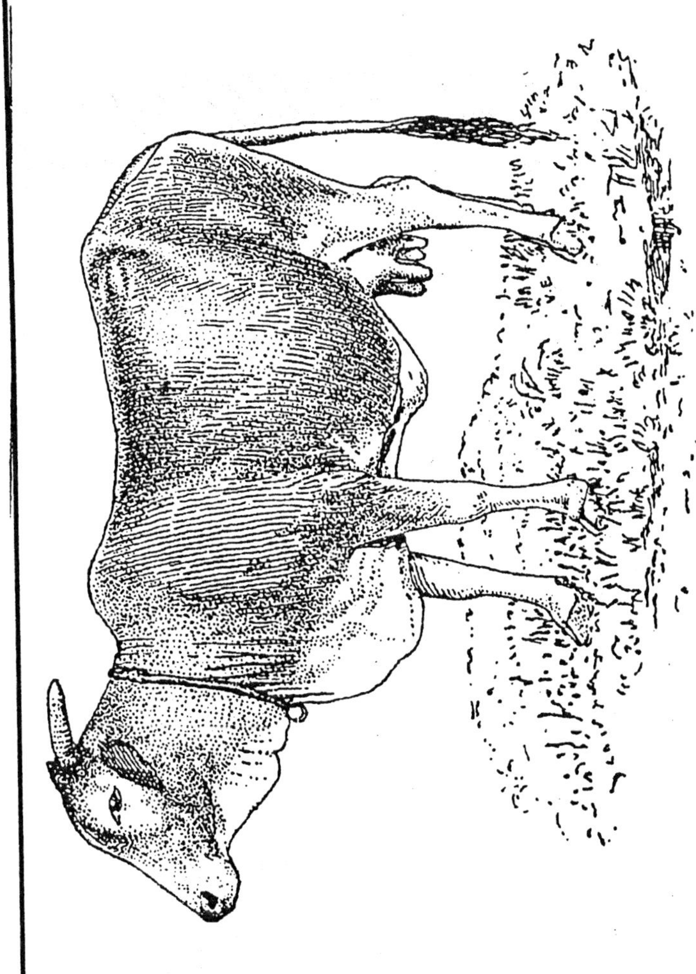

Fig. 3: Montgomery Cow

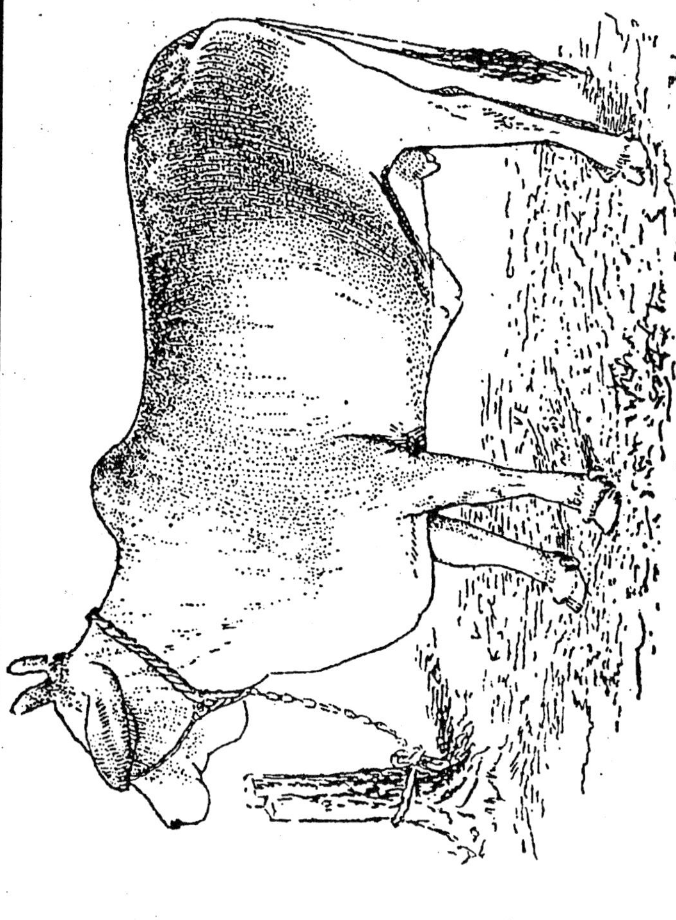

Fig. 4: Montgomery Cow

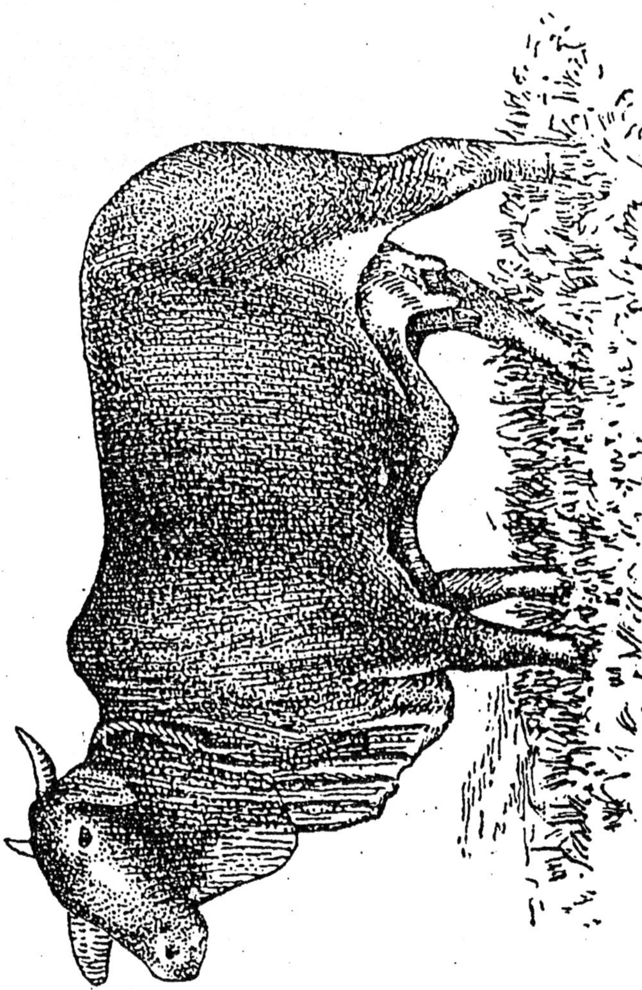

Fig. 5: Montgomery Cow "Hoosni" Pusa Herd. Yield During Last-Lactation Period (11 months), 5,470 lb.

female, are well developed; the frame is long, deep, massive, and is supported on short, well set legs; long, level quarters; deep, muscular thighs; wide loins; the hind part more developed than the fore; generally mild-tempered; the colour varies-there are, reds, blacks, greys, whites, and spotted. They are most symmetrical and beautiful animals. The cows have large udders and well-shaped, fairly large, regularly placed teats. These cows give from twenty to thirty-two pounds of milk a day when in full milk, and yield milk from eight to ten months at a time. Some give a good deal more. They are very hardy and stand the change of climate well if properly looked after. These fine cattle are taken in large numbers to Kolkata and other cities and towns for sale. The price of good cows in their own districts is from Rs. 80 to Rs. 120, but in Kolkata they fetch from Rs. 200 to Rs. 300 each or more according to the demand and supply.

Sind Cattle

There is some similarity of type between Montgomery cattle and those bred in Lower Sind. In all probability they are strains from the common stock and resemble each other excepting in size, in colour, and looks, but are equally good as milkers, and fetch equally high prices. These are the two most valuable breeds of milch cows in India. Their milk is rich in butter fat when compared with those of other Indian and continental breeds.

Hansi or Hissar

Hisaar and Hansi are neighbouring districts in the section of the Punjab called Haryana. The breed of cattle found in these districts is thought a great deal of. They stand from 56 to 64 inches high; their heads are light; faces long; ears are long and incline to be pendulous; necks short; humps high; hips broad and hindquarters square; udders and teats large; they carry their heads erect, and have long, curved horns inclined inwards and backwards, and thin, long tails; they are of great substance and have long bodies, deep wide chests, and massive and rather short legs fairly apart to support the frame; feet small, hard, and well-shaped. The dewlap is large and pendulous; the sheath in the male is short and close. The bullocks are very big and strong and draw great weights and heavy ploughs, but are not so fast as bullocks of some other breeds. They are generally of a nice white or grey colour, but sometimes red, black, brown, or piebald ones are found. These cattle are exceedingly handsome.

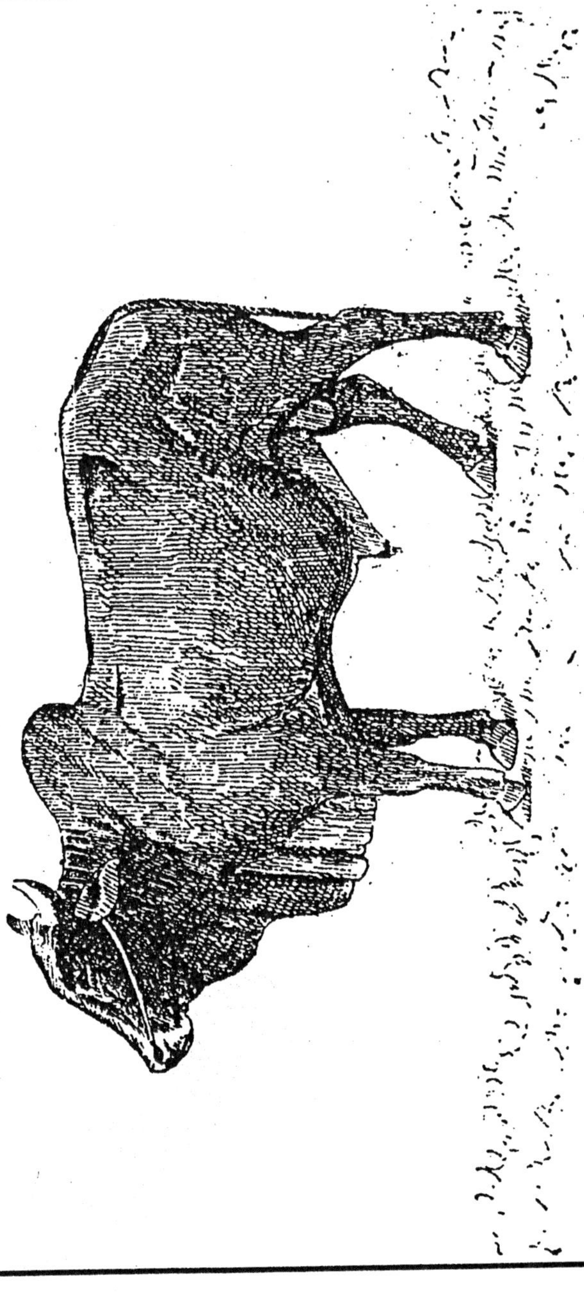

Fig. 6: Sind Bull at Kirkee Farm Herd.

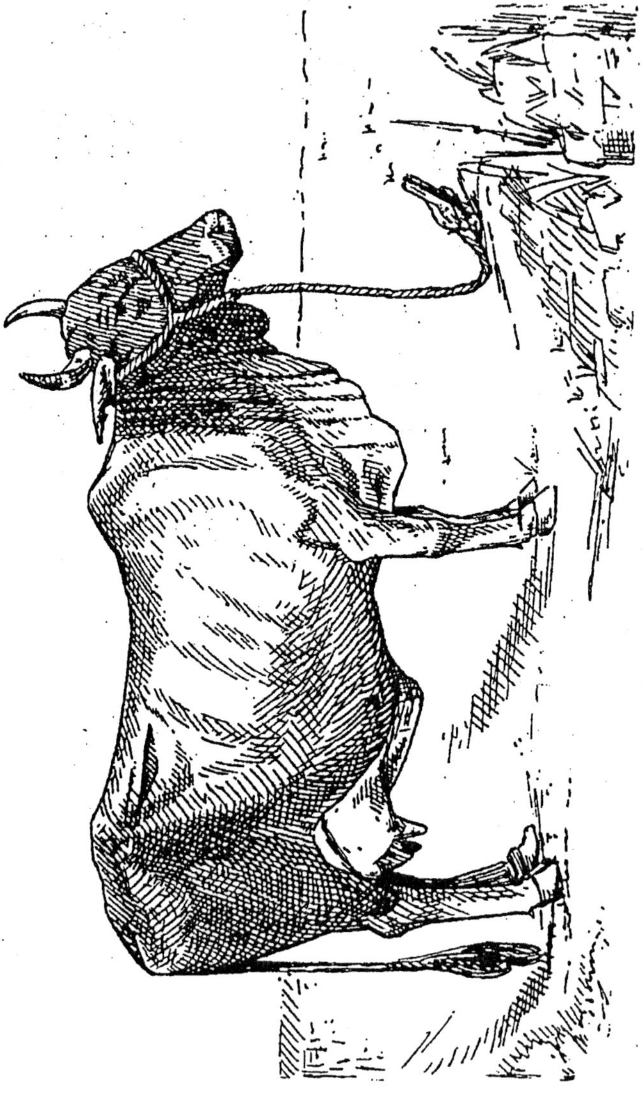

Fig. 7: Sind Cow at Kirkee Farm Herd.

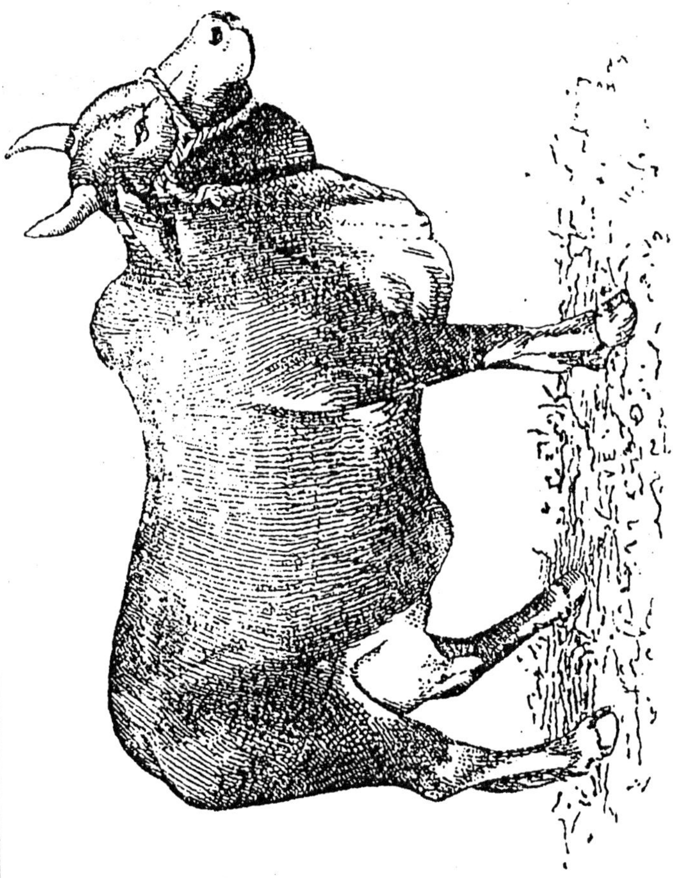

Fig. 8: Sind Cow

In their own districts the cows give from twenty to thirty-two pounds of milk in twenty-four hours, but when removed from the fine pasturage of Hissar their milk somewhat decreases. The milk is of the best quality, generally of a creamy white colour.

In their own districts these cows sell from Rs. 80 to Rs. 150 each, and the bullocks from Rs. 100 to Rs. 150 each. In Kolkata they will sell for double the above prices.

Nagaur

The Nagauri cattle are said to be natives of Nagaur, in Bikaner-Rajputana. In former days they were largely bred at Delhi, and were seen all over the North-West and Central Provinces.

The cows are very gentle, and, some of the best give from twenty to thirty pounds of milk a day, but the milk is not very rich. The majority do not give as such as the Hansi does.

Nagauri cattle are of the well-known trotting breed; the bullocks are much prized, and were formerly used by Indian gentlemen for their carriages. More than half a century ago they were extensively used in large cities by rich Indians, and in those days were carefully bred for the purpose; but now they are not so well preserved, and good cattle are very scarce.

Some of these cattle are very tall and narrow; the tallest measure 64 inches in height. They have curved horns, long and narrow heads, and a round humps tands out between their horns; their humps are high and narrow; their hind-quarters are narrow; their tails are long and thin, with a thick and long bunch of black, silky hair on the end. Their hoofs and pasterns are long, and their thin body enables them to trot so well. They are not very fleshy, lacking the great substance of the Hissar breed. The pace of these bullocks is nearly equal to that of a good trotting horse, but they are not able to draw heavy burdens; their carriages are much like light ekkas, with two wheels, and pole tilted up to prevent any weight falling on the neck of the bullocks.

They are white in colour, and are the most delicate cattle in India. Like the Hansi, they are not very prolific.

Good cows of the pure breed sell from Rs. 100 to Rs. 200 each, and good trotting bullocks from Rs. 200 to Rs. 300 each.

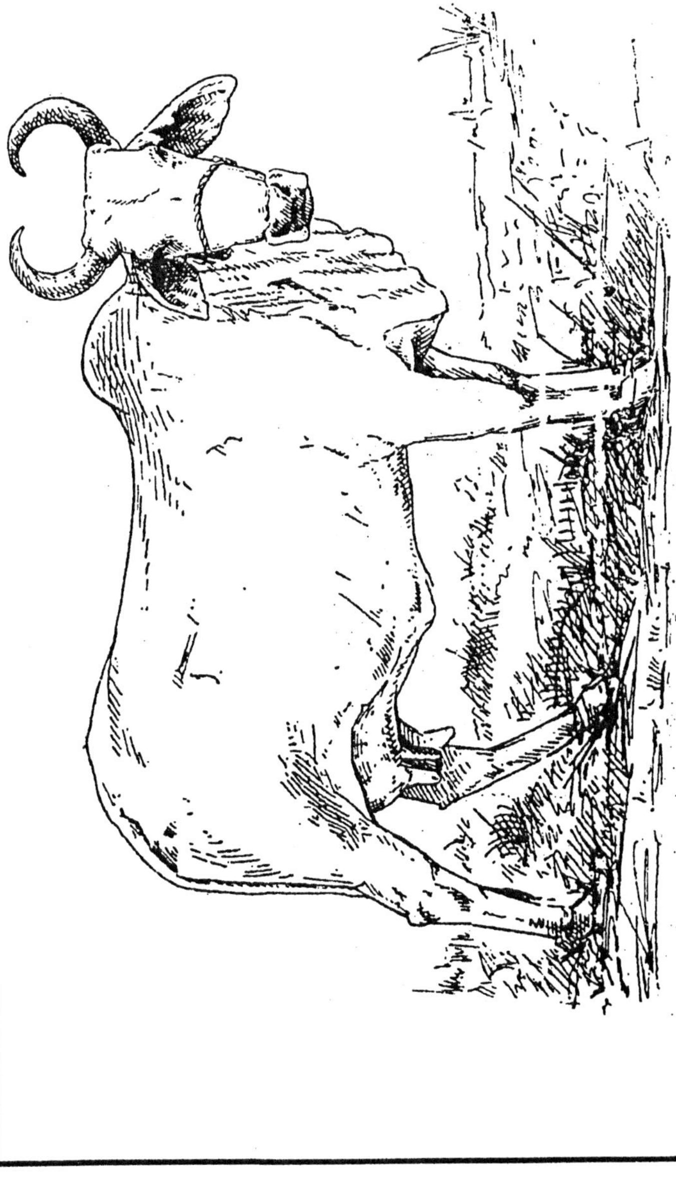

Fig. 9: Hissar Cow

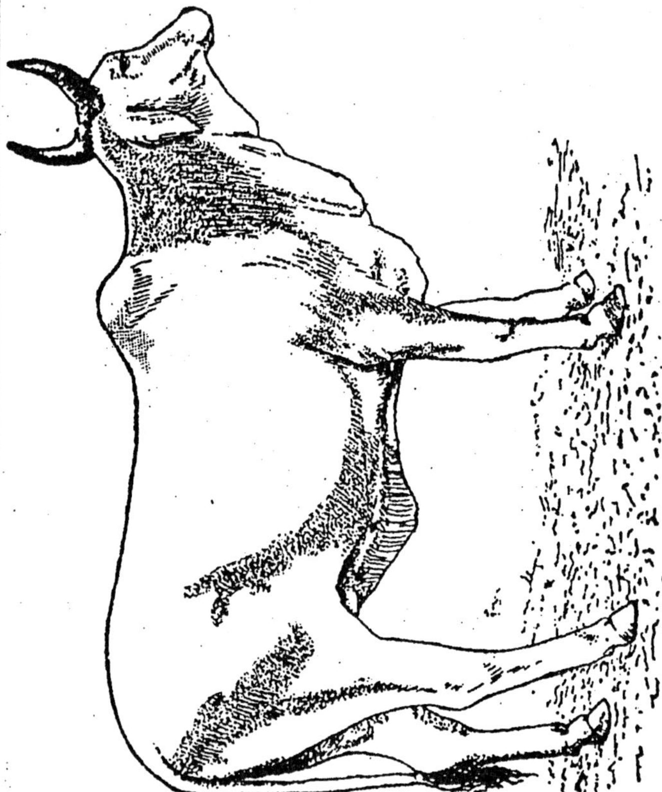

Fig. 10: Hansi Cow at Hissar Farm

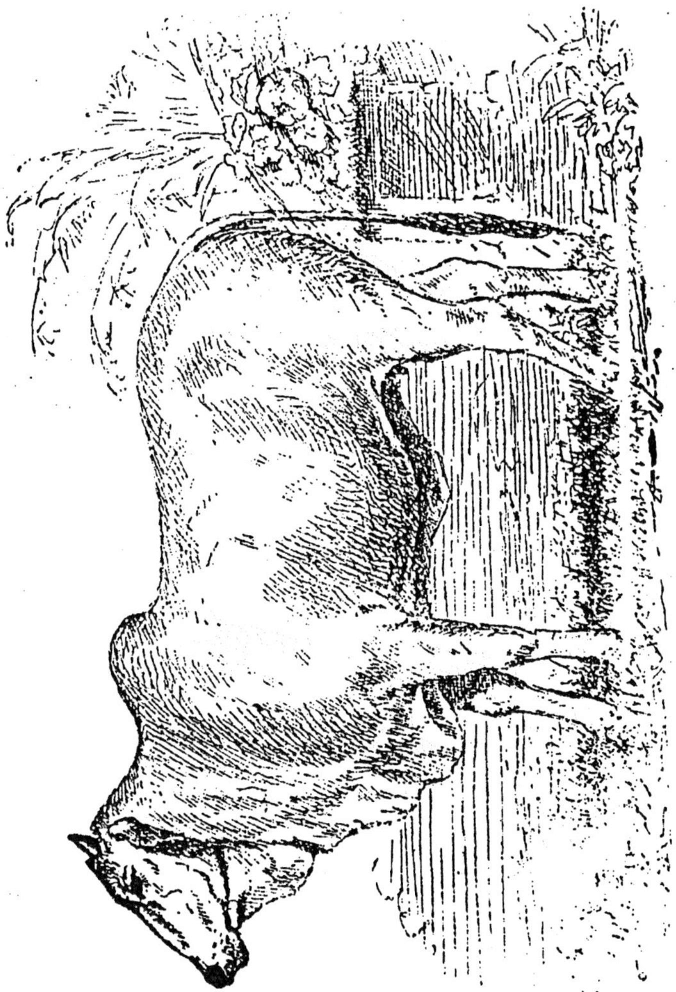

Fig. 11: Hansi Heifer

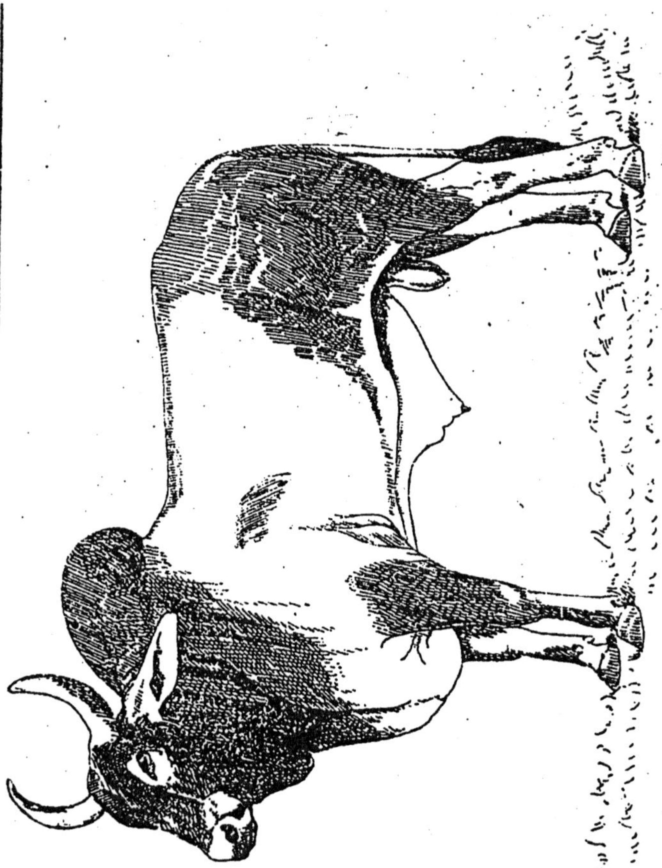

Fig. 12: Hansi Bull at Hissar Farm

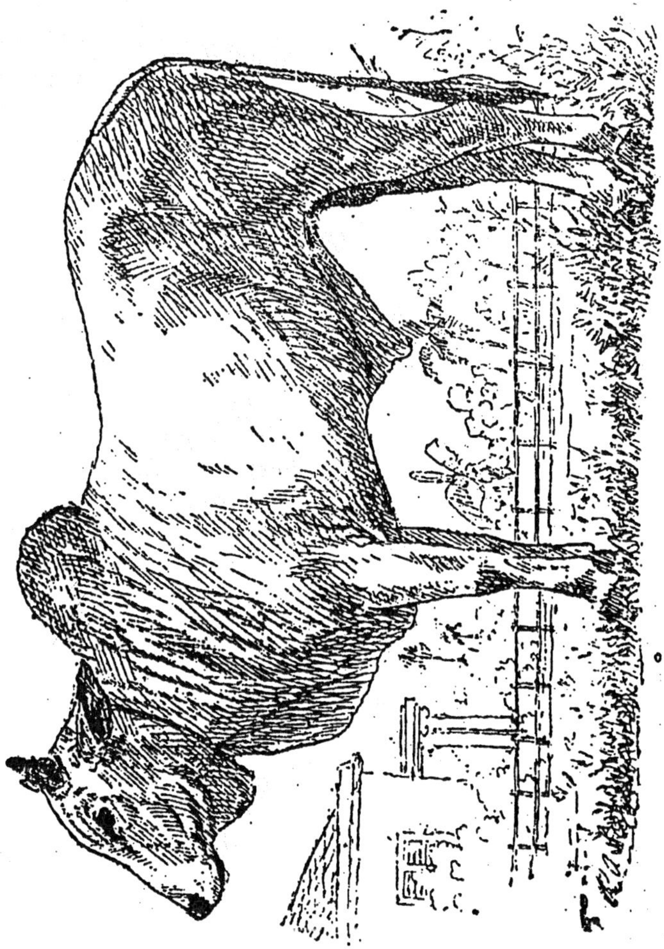

Fig. 13: Young Hansi Bull

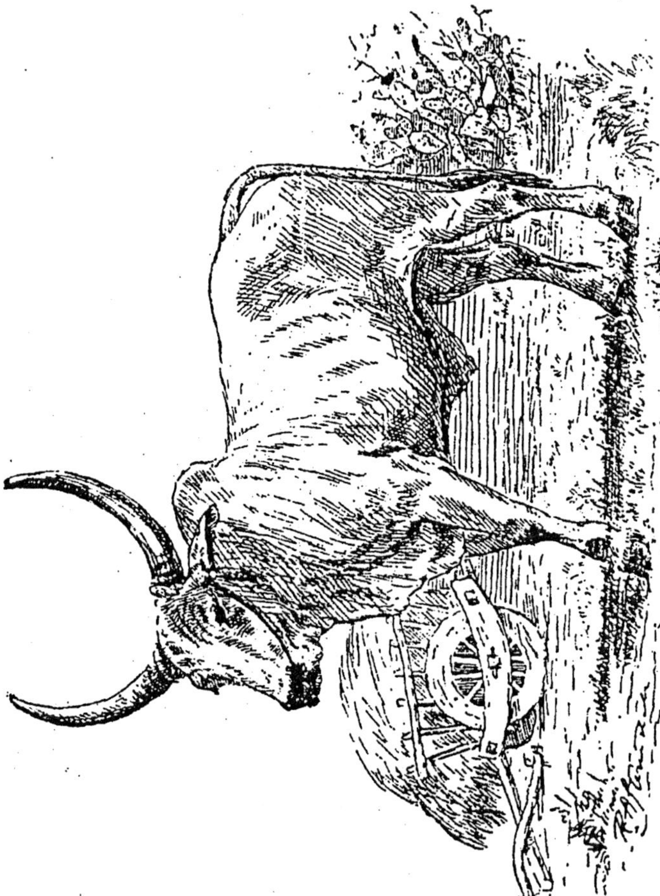

Fig. 14: Hansi Bullock from Hissar Farm

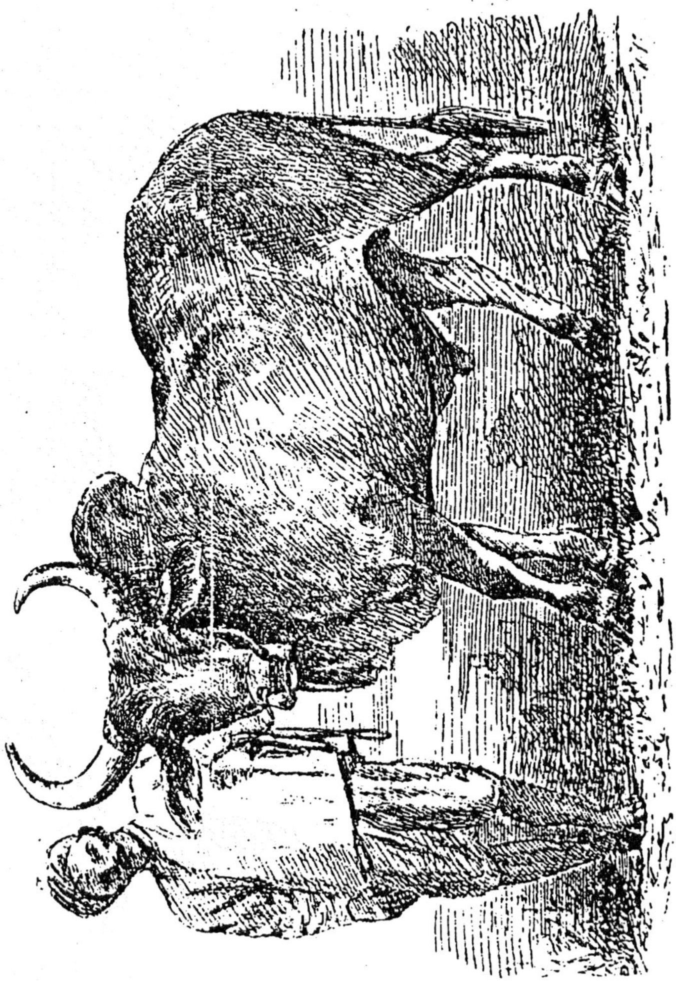

Fig. 15: Hansi Bullock

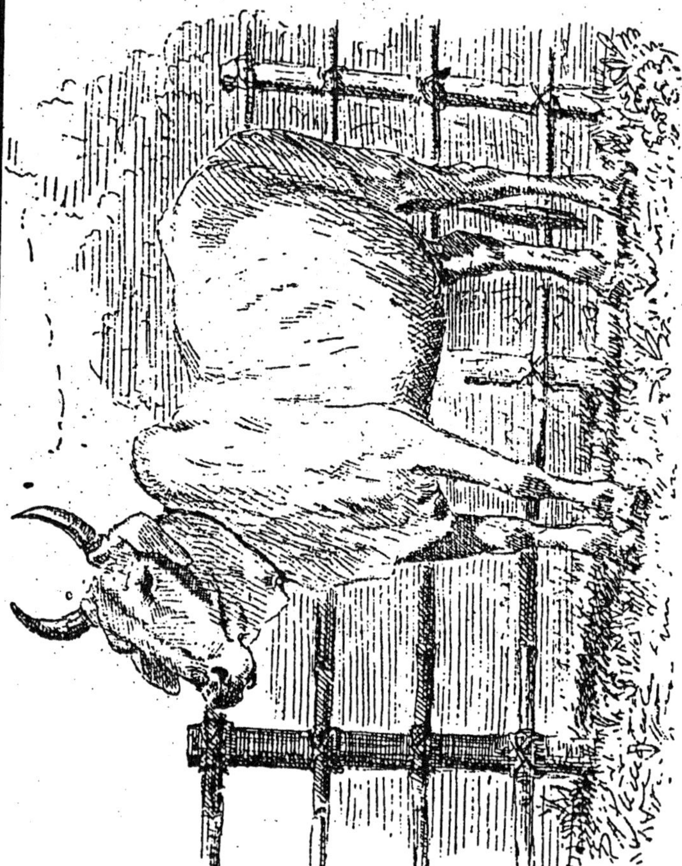

Fig. 16: Cross Hansi Country

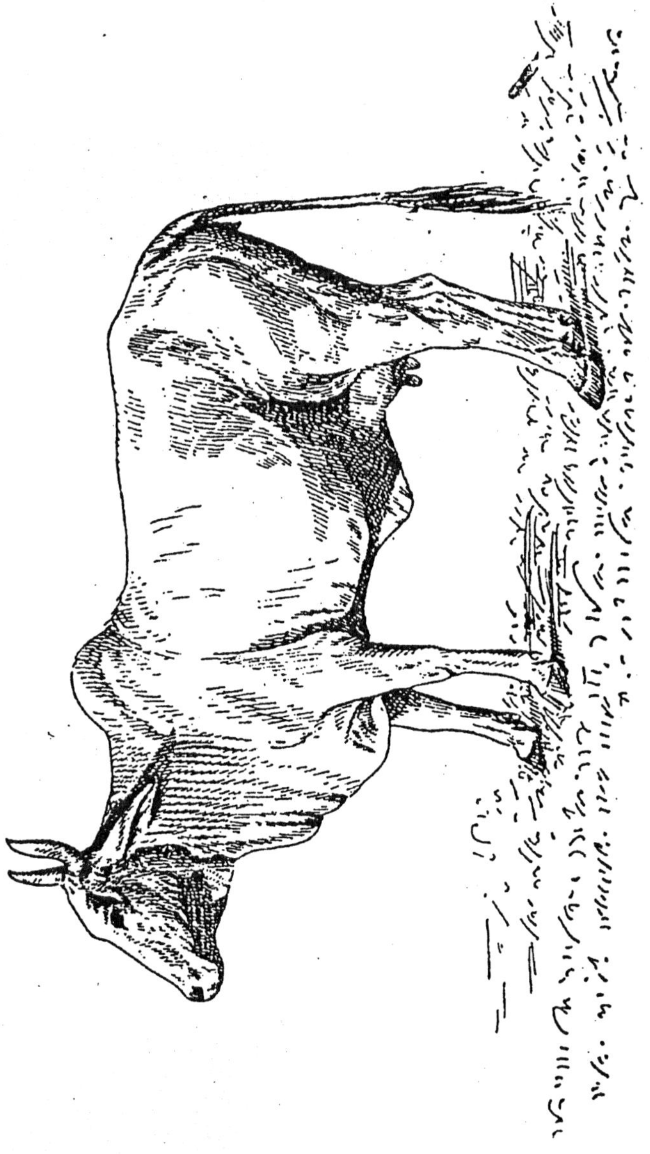

Fig. 17: Nagauri Cow–Bred in Barmer. Taken at Jodhpur

Nellore or Ongole

Nellore and Ongole are in the Madras Presidency. This breed has long been celebrated for the milking qualities of the cows, and the great strength and spirit of endurance of the bullocks, on account of which they fetch large prices.

A good specimen of the Nellore breed is a huge animal standing from 60 to 64 inches in height, with a noble look, and very gentle and slow in its movements. It is readily recognized by its form and horns. The horns are hardly over longer than from three to nine inches, and are tapering to a blunt point; the animal has a dull countenance and large, prominent and heavy-loosing eyes; its face is short and its forehead and muzzle broad; its ears are large and lopping; its eyes, hoof, and tail tuft are black; it carries its head erect, and has a short stout neck, rising over the withers into a huge hump which frequently inclines to one side; its back is short and straight; its chest is fairly deep and wide, and its frame compact and solid-looking, with a heavy dewlap; its legs are clean and massive, straight and fairly apart to support the body; its skin is fine and covered with soft, short hair. The prevailing colour is white, and black and white.

Cattle of this breed generally are heavy-looking creatures, but there is a tendency in some of them to grow tall and leggy. The bullocks (a pair of them) draw thirty maunds in a cart, and are excellent for the plough.

The price of a pair of good bullocks ranges from Rs. 250 to Rs. 500. The cows give from twenty to twenty-eight pounds of milk a day. The milk is very rich. Good cows sell for from Rs. 100 to Rs. 300 each.

Gir

Sometimes called Kathiawar. Gir is in the Mumbai Presidency. This breed of cattle is of medium height, of good form and substance, and the cows give from sixteen to twenty-four pounds of milk a day. They have smaller horns and larger ears than the Hansi, and not very large humps. The colour is usually a mixture of red and white or black and white. The head, horns and ears are specially characteristic. The frontal bones are well developed and very prominent. The ears are long and pendulous, broader at the end than at the root. They are rather nervous and irritable in temper, and

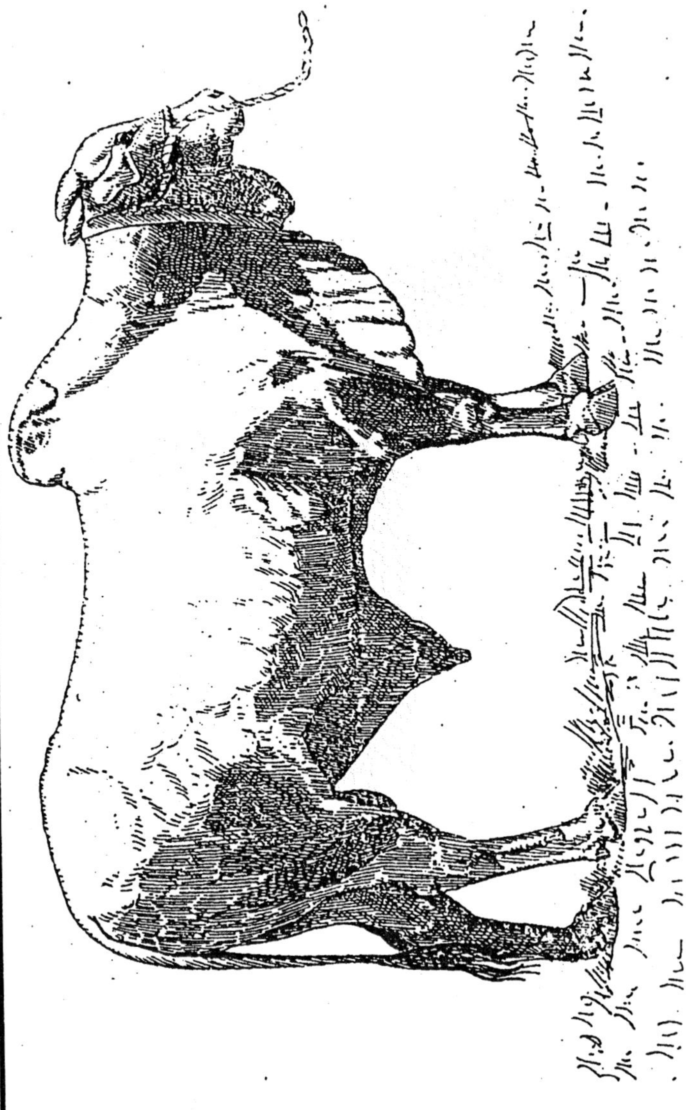

Fig. 18: First Prize–Brahmani Bull, Ongole Breed

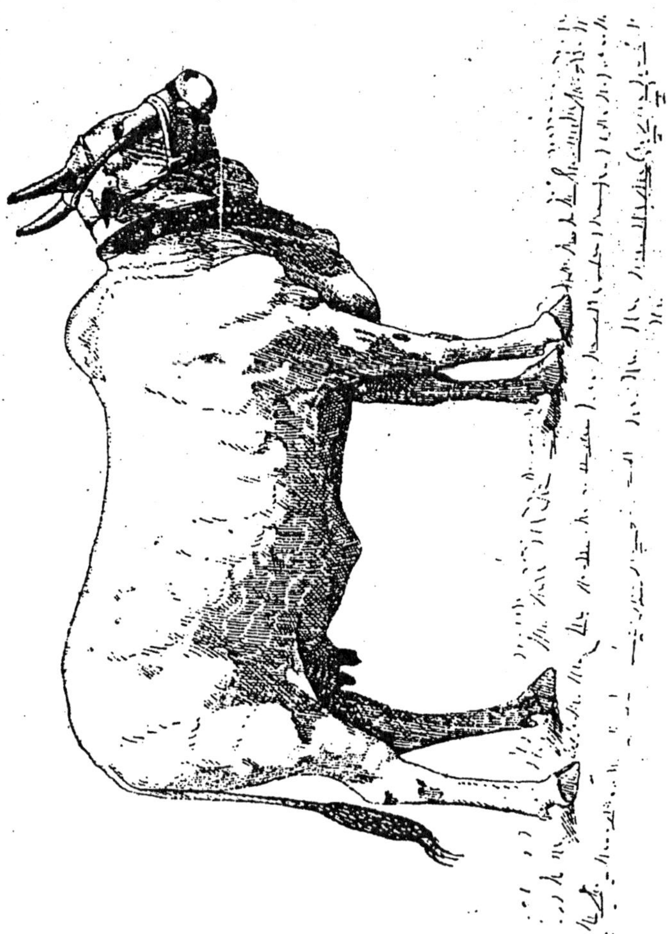

Fig. 19: First Prize–Ongole Cow

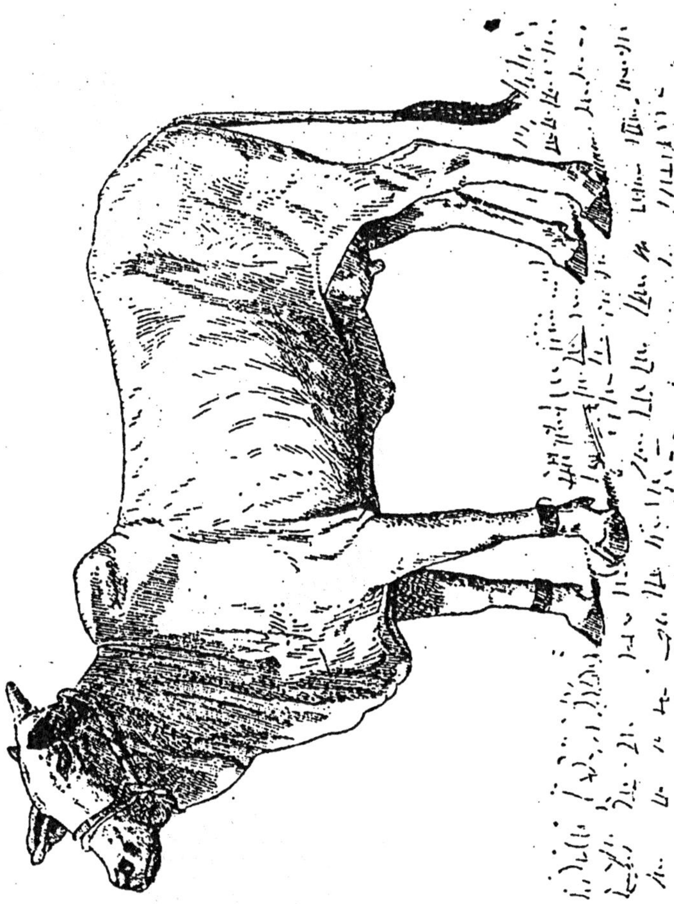

Fig. 20: Ongole Heifer

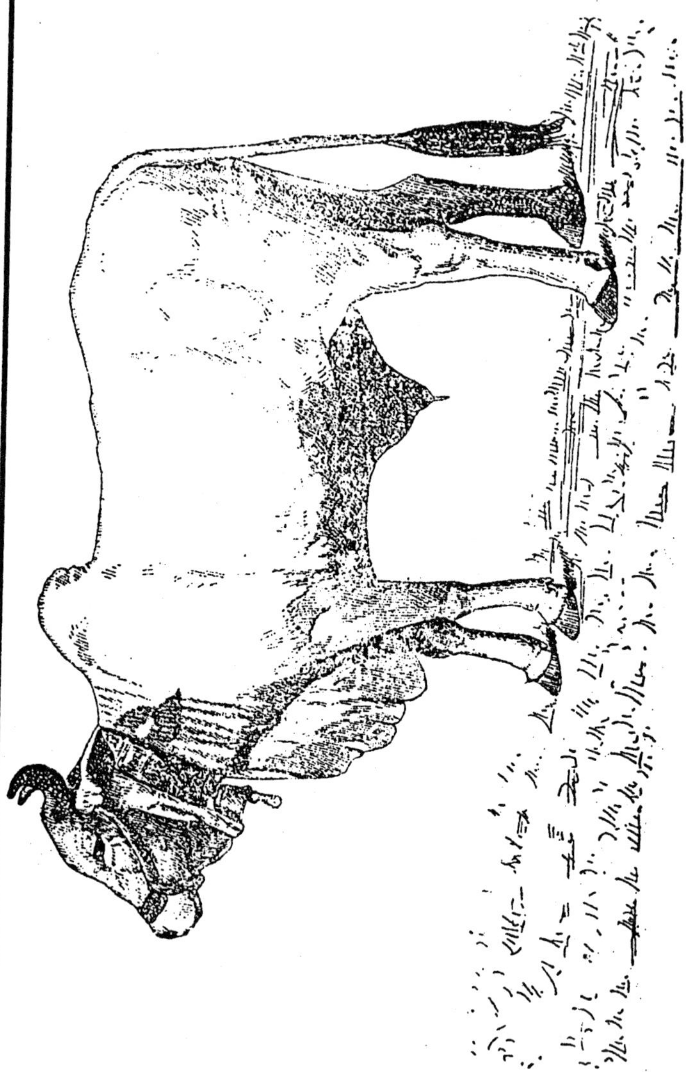

Fig. 21: Prize–Ongole Bullock

the cows are not as persistent and regular milkers as the Montgomery or Sind. They are considered the best milk breed in the Mumbai Presidency.

The bullocks are large, strong, and heavy, and do well in the plough, and draw heavy burdens. These cattle sell for from Rs. 60 to Rs. 150 each.

Kankreji Cattle

This is another good breed of the Mumbai Presidency. They are tall, substantial active, and docile. The bullocks are good in the cart and plough, and are highly prized. The cows are fair milkers, a few have given as much as 4,000 pounds at one lactation. Good cattle of this breed are expensive. They are very seldom seen outside of their Presidency. The Gir and Kankreji are the two principal breeds of the Presidency.

The Kankreji breed is also called Guzarathi, but the breed most common in Gujarat is a cross between the Gir and other breeds.

Goorgaira, in the Mooltan district, produces another good breed of cattle. The cows have all the good qualities of the Hissar, but are not so large or so delicate as the latter. They are middle-sized and handsome, broad and well-knit, and of a dark colour. Some of the best have black points. They are somewhat of the type of the Montgomery, and are probably a cross between Montgomery bulls and the cows of the district. They are hardy and healthy, and beautiful milkers. Their horns are not very long.

A cow gives from sixteen to twenty pounds of milk a day, and fetches from Rs. 100 to Rs. 150 in her own district.

Mooltan and Amritsar Cows

Large number of Montgomery cattle have been brought to the Mooltan and Amritsar districts and are kept pure and bred by the people. Some are crossed with the local cattle. Those that are kept pure retain all the good characteristics of the breed, but those that are mixed show a variety of types. The cows from these districts are brought in large numbers to Kolkata and other large towns and cities and sold for from Rs. 200 to Rs. 250 each. Many of them are very good milkers, and hardy and healthy when given proper care. In their own districts they sell for from Rs. 100 to Rs. 140 each.

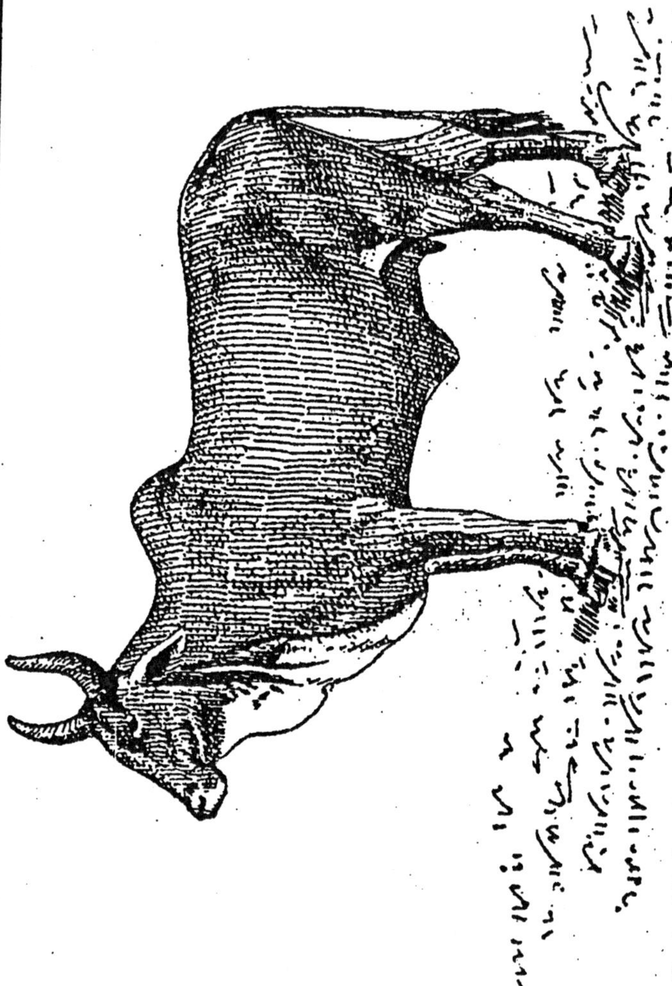

Fig. 22: Typical Gujrat Cow of the Best Sort for Breeding, taken at Patri–Kankreji Breed of Mature Age

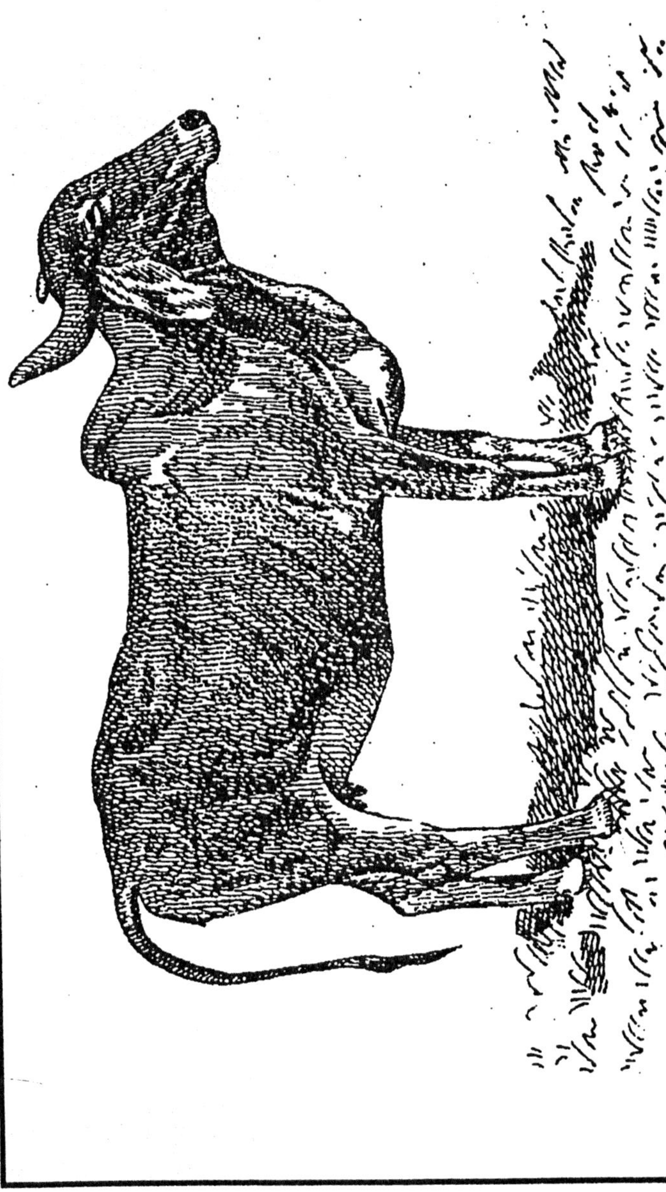

Fig. 23: Gir (Kathiawar) Cow—Colour Red. Patri

Krishna Valley Cattle

This is another breed of fairly good cattle. They are medium-sized and well-built. The bullocks are good workers, but the cows are not good milkers.

Kangayam

There are two varieties of these cattle: one is large and other small. The cows of the large variety are fairly good milkers, and can be bought in their own districts for Rs. 40 to Rs. 60 each. They are a local breed. Kangayam is in Southern India.

Mysore Bullocks

Besides the above-mentioned principal breeds of milk and draught cattle, the Amrit Mahal breed of Mysore produces excellent bullocks, but the cows are not good milker; they rarely give more than four to six pounds of milk a day.

These bullocks are noted for their great strength and powers of endurance. They rarely exceed 60 inches in height, and generally are only about 48 inches; but in proportion to their size they are remarkably deep and wide in the chest, long and broad in the back, round in the barrel, well ribbed up, and strong in the shoulders and limbs.

They are active and fiery, and some of them walk faster than the troops; they generally have straight horns from two to three feet in length, tapering and sharp-pointed, inclining forward, and slightly approaching each other at the top; their countenance is sprightly; their eyes are large, black and prominent, expressive and full of fire; they have long and moderately narrow faces; their muzzles and hoofs are black; they carry their heads erect on a moderately-sized and well-formed neck, they have fair-sized humps and small dewlaps. The cows are generally white, but the bulls are grey; some are dark-coloured.

A good bullock will fetch from Rs. 100 to Rs. 200 in its own district.

Dhanni Cattle

This breed of cattle is known as Pothwar and Nukra, and is confined to the Jhelum, Attock, and Rawalpindi districts. The bullocks are large and handsome, very strong and good workers,

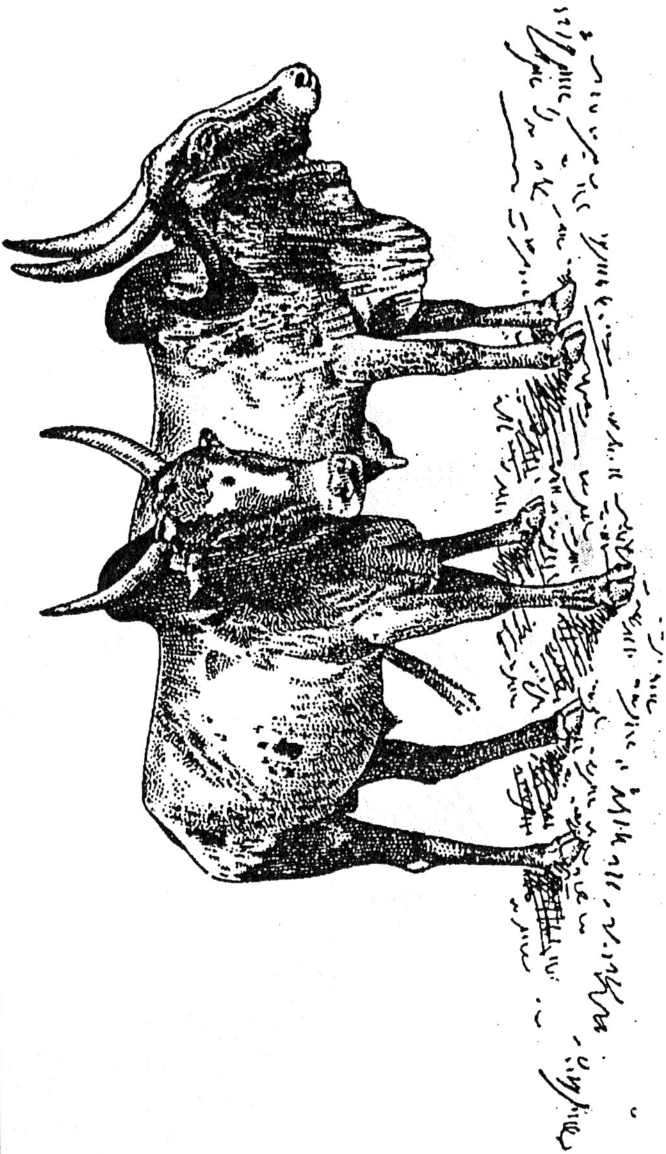

Fig. 24: Pair or Amrit Mahal Bullocks

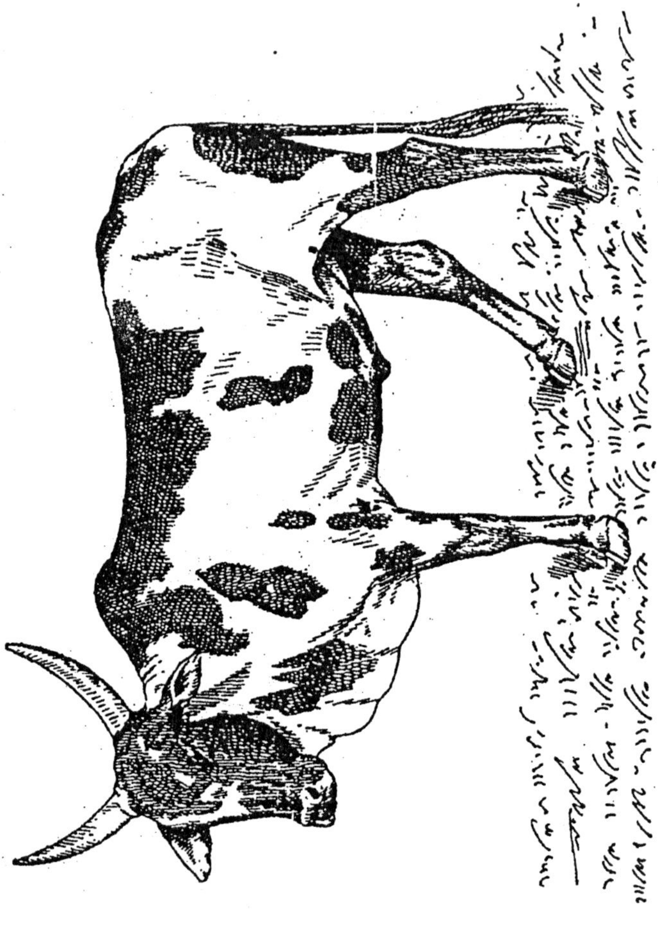

Fig. 25: Mysore-Nadu Bull, Common Variety

but the cows are neglected and small and do not give much milk, though some large and good milkers are found among them. If they were properly fed and cared for they would be a valuable breed. The bullocks are 50 to 56 inches high.

Awankari Breed

This beautiful breed of cattle is found in North Punjab. The bullocks are from 48 to 60 inches in height; well proportioned and strong; usually black and white in colour; the cows are fairly good milkers. They cost from Rs. 100 to Rs. 150 each in their own country.

Bengal Cattle

In Bengal there is no special breed of good cattle. The best specimens are cross-breeds between cows of the district and bulls of the Hissar, Montgomery, Shahabad or other breeds.

A few years ago some Hissar and Mostgomery bulls were brought to Burdwan and Birbhoom in order to improve the local cattle. But not many of the zamindars or ryots appreciated this, and when the bulls died, no efforts were made to import new ones.

In different parts of the country some rich zamindars have imported a few pure-bred or half-bred bulls and let them loose as Brahmani bulls. The animals roam about all over the place, and the people are allowed their services; but nowadays people are gradually getting eager to improve their cattle and this system should be reintroduced with advantage.

The Local and District Boards should take up this matter and import good Montgomery, Sind, Mooltan, and Shahabad bulls into all the districts of Bengal, where improvement of cattle is possible. Every village or group of villages should be induced to maintain and keep one or more bulls, and the people should be encouraged to improve their cattle by offering them prizes for the best specimens of milch cows and home-bred calves. Prizes should not be given for bullocks, as they are generally imported from other parts of the country.

Now as each Province is provided with its Live Stock Expert-solution of this problem can be expected in the near future after the situation has been studied by him. All common, old and weakly bulls should be either castrated or removed from the village. The best male and female calves should be properly fed and cared for. If

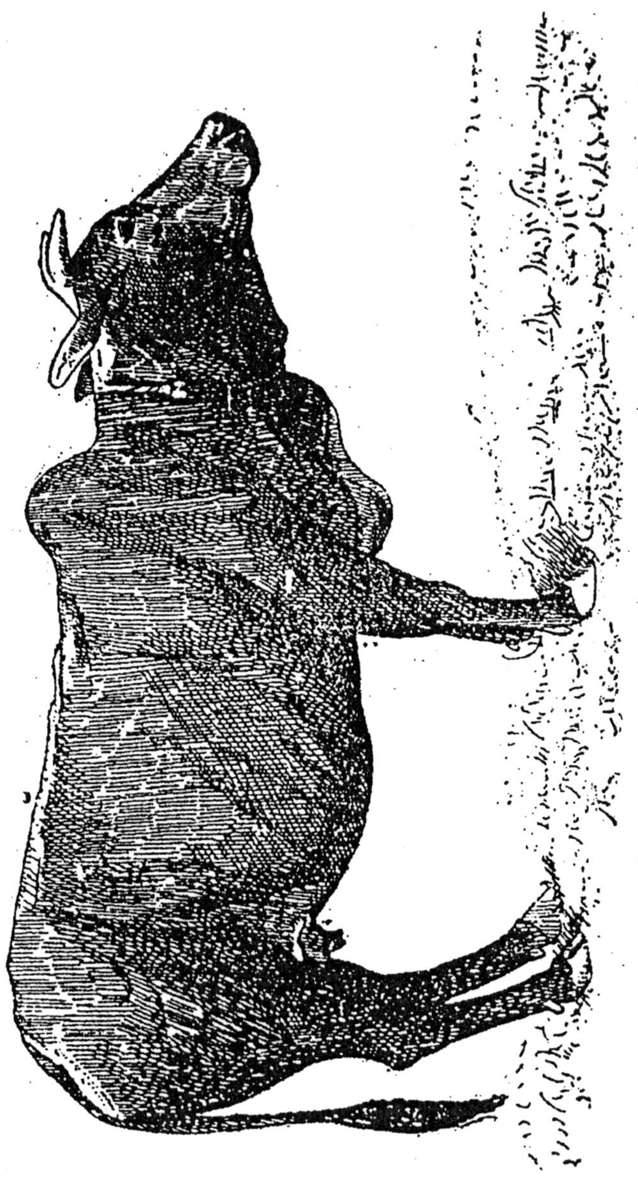

Fig. 26: Better Class Bengali Cow

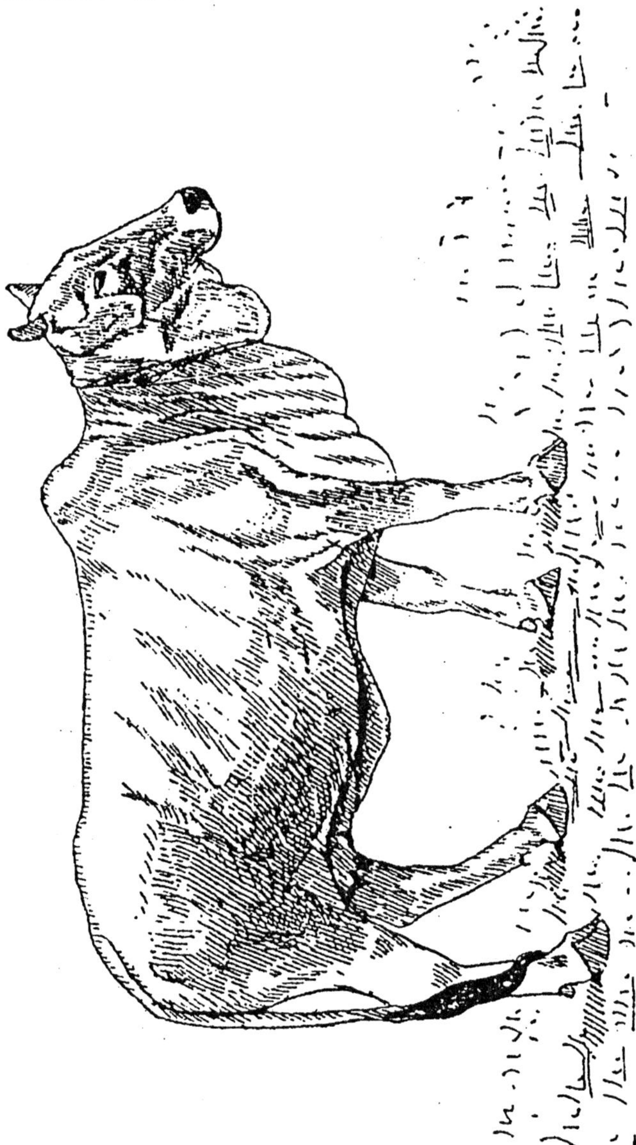

Fig. 27: Better Class Shahabad Cow

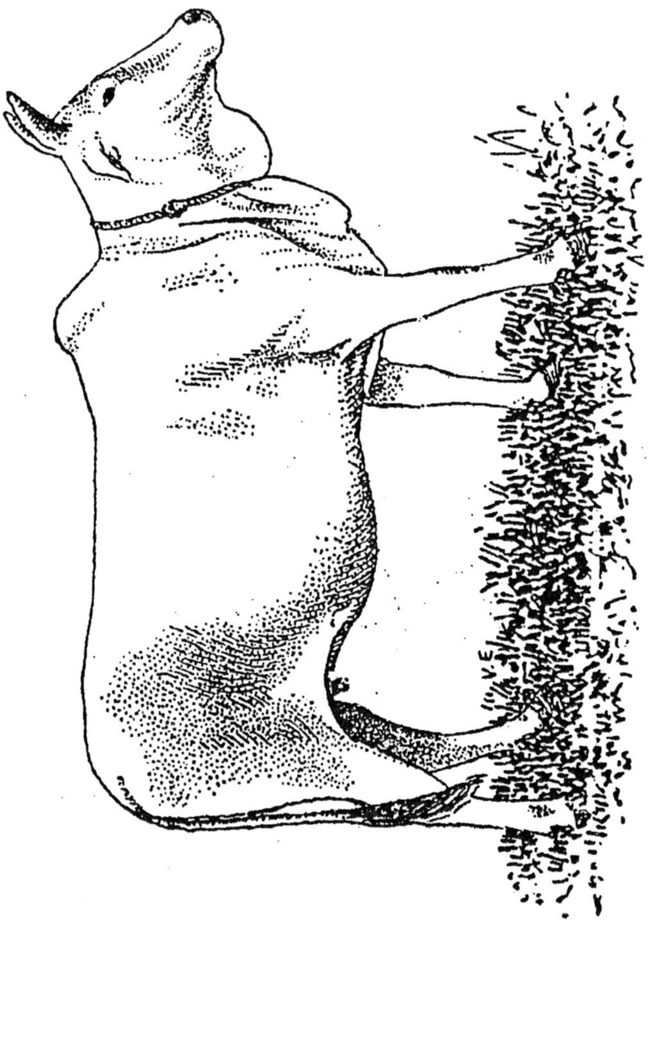

Fig. 28: Better Class Shahabad Cow

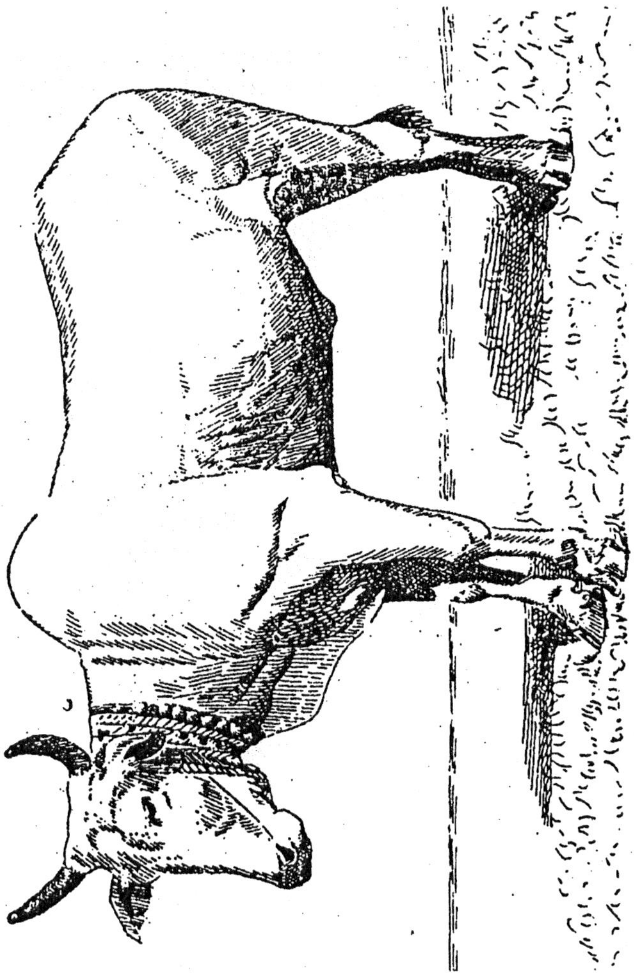

Fig. 29: Shahabad Bullock

this plan were adopted throughout Bengal, in five years there would be a very marked improvement in the cattle.

In Kolkata there are very few pedigreed pulls, but a number of half-bred ones are kept for breeding purposes.

The best bullocks for the plough and cart in Bengal are the cross-bred between the better class country cows and Sitamari, Montgomery or Sindhi bulls. A large number of bullocks are also imported from Shahabad.

Up-country cattle generally deteriorate very much in Bengal on account of the climate and change of food specially during the rainy seasons, when mosquitoes are in abundance and there is scarcity of green fodder. The rich and educated Bengalis and Marwaris allow their cows to grow fat by injudicious feeding; the ignorant and poor Bengalis in this matter cannot afford to take proper care of their cows and calves for want of men and money. Large up-country cattle are too delicate and need much more care than the ordinary. Cross-bred bullocks are strong and hardy, and the people prefer them for the plough and cart.

Cross-bred cows are found all over Bengal. Some of them are excellent milkers for their size, and are more hardy than the pure breed. They sell generally for less than half the price of cows of pure blood.

A half-bred Bengali cow will give from ten to fourteen pounds of milk a day, and will sell for from Rs. 80 to Rs. 150. A half-bred bullock will stand about 48 to 50 inches high, and will sell for from Rs. 150 to Rs. 250 per pair.

The ordinary Bengali cattle are very small and weak, measuring from 32 to 40 inches in height, and sell for from Rs. 20 to Rs. 50 each. The bullocks cannot do much in the cart or at the plough, and the cows give on an average from one to four pounds of milk a day.

Bihar Cattle

The best breed of cattle in Bihar is found in the Shahabad district. The prevailing colour is grey. The head is carried fairly erect, is long, and tapers to the nose. The forehead is broad and slightly convex. The eyes are deep-set and mild. The horns are short, thick, and blunt at the point. They are from 45 to 54 inches high. The neck is short and thick, and the dewlap of medium size. The back rises a little towards the loins; the loins are broad and the quarters are sloping. The shoulders are well defined; the legs are well proportioned with good bone and carried well apart. In the cow the udder is well developed with the teats properly separated and the milk vein is distinctly prominent. The hoofs and horns are black and hard. The animals have a well-bred appearance. The best cows give from twelve to sixteen pounds of milk a day and cost from Rs. 120 to Rs. 170 each.

The bullocks are very good in the cart and at the plough. They fetch as much as from Rs. 200 to Rs. 300 a pair. Good bulls of this breed would do very well to cross with small Bengali cows.

All through Bihar one will find good cross-bred cows. European planters and some rich landlords have imported English, Montgomery, and Hissar bulls to improve the cattle of their locality.

Bhagalpore Cattle

These cattle are not thought much of. The bullocks are usually leggy and flat-sided and the cows are poor milkers. They do not do well in most parts of Bengal.

Darjeeling Cattle

There are three distinct breeds of cattle met with in Darjeeling District, *viz.*, (1) "Siri" breed, said to be imported from Bhutan, the word "Siri " is derived from the Sanskrit word "Sree" or "Sri" meaning handsome; (2) the "Nepali" or "Pahari" breed, these are the real pahari or hill cattle of the district, they were originally introduced from Nepal; (3) the ordinary "Zebu plains breed," found in the Terai.

A species of wild cattle the "Mithun," also called "'Gayal," is occasionally seen domesticated and buffaloes are also to be met with. The above are indigenous to the district, but in addition English and Australian breeds have been introduced with a view to improve the milk supply but attempts to breed from them are not very hopeful, although much liked by paharis. The Siri cows are of good size and shape and have large udders and give generally from 4 to 6 or 7 seers of very rich milk. The bullocks are very hardy and stand the climate well. The Nepali or Pahari breeds are diminutive and the cows are not much liked by the gowallas owing to the small amount of milk yield, they are like the Siris very hardy and just the animal

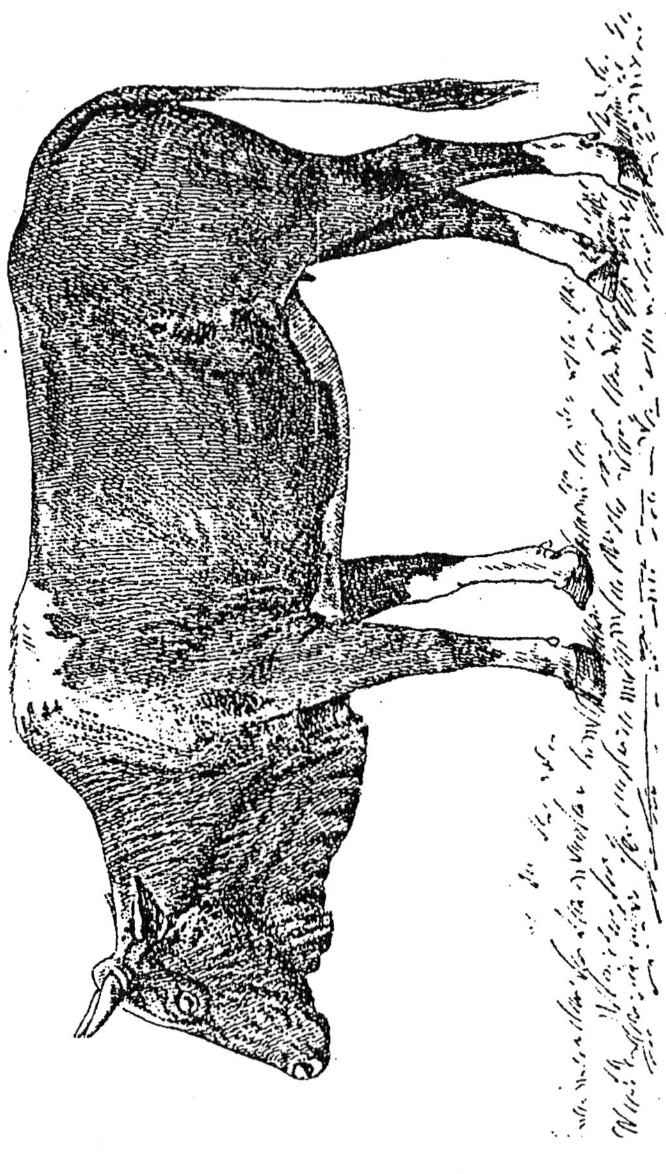

Fig. 30: Pure Siri Cow

suited to the country. The cross breeds are not so hardy and require great care and attention, and will not thrive on forest grazing alone, although they are good milkers.

Patna Cattle

There was a breed of cattle in the Patna and Bankipore districts called the Taylor breed. Many years ago Mr. Taylor, the Commissioner of the district, imported some Australian bulls and crossed the local cows by them. This has produced some very good milkers. But the cows and bullocks in these districts are small, light in build, and red or brown in colour. Some of the cows used to give from twenty-four to thirty-six pounds of milk in twenty-four hours, but the majority give only from twelve to sixteen pounds of milk a day. These cattle have in a great measure deteriorated as they were not stable breeds. The bullocks do not do well at work, as they are not large or strong and do not stand the heat well. Cows that give from twenty to thirty pounds of milk a day can be bought for from Rs. 150 to Rs. 250 each. This breed is not much seen nowadays.

English and Australian Cattle are not a success in India. They suffer much from the heat and damp, and the milk greatly decreases; not many are able to give them the care and attention they need. Nevertheless, some people prefer them to Indian cows. If a person has a large cool house and a few biggahs of land with many trees and a tank on it, and can afford an attendant for each cow, then he may keep them successfully.

They do not suffer so much in the hills. Some cows have done well on the plains for a year or two, and then suddenly died after a short illness; others have died in the first year. They are highly susceptible to foot-and-mouth, rinderpest, and other infectious diseases common to cattle in this country, and few survive.

They need to be fed on the same kind of food they have been accustomed to in their native land but the change should be gradual. Any sudden change in food or treatment will prove injurious. Mustard-seed oilcake should never be given. Linseed, tilseed, groundnut and cocoanut oilcake are good for them. They should have plenty of green food. Many look upon English cows in India as a very troublesome and costly luxury.

Cross-Breed English Cows are found all over India, especially in Madras, parts of Mumbai, the North-West Provinces, Bengal, and

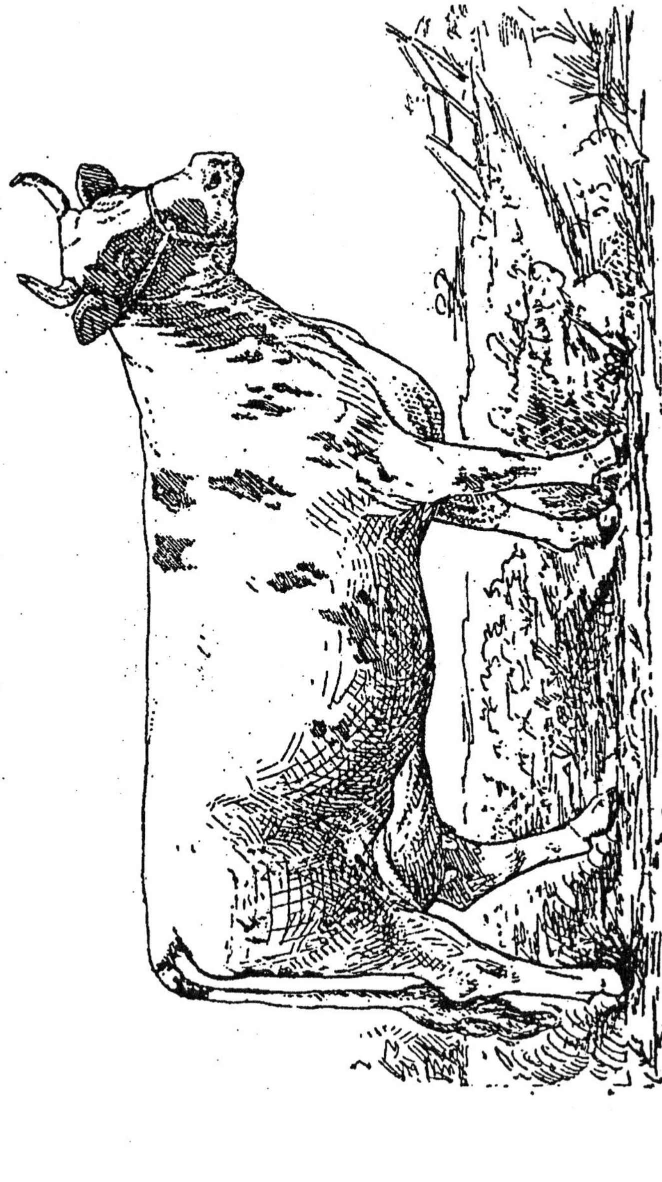

Fig. 31: Ayrshire Cow, Dewdrop I

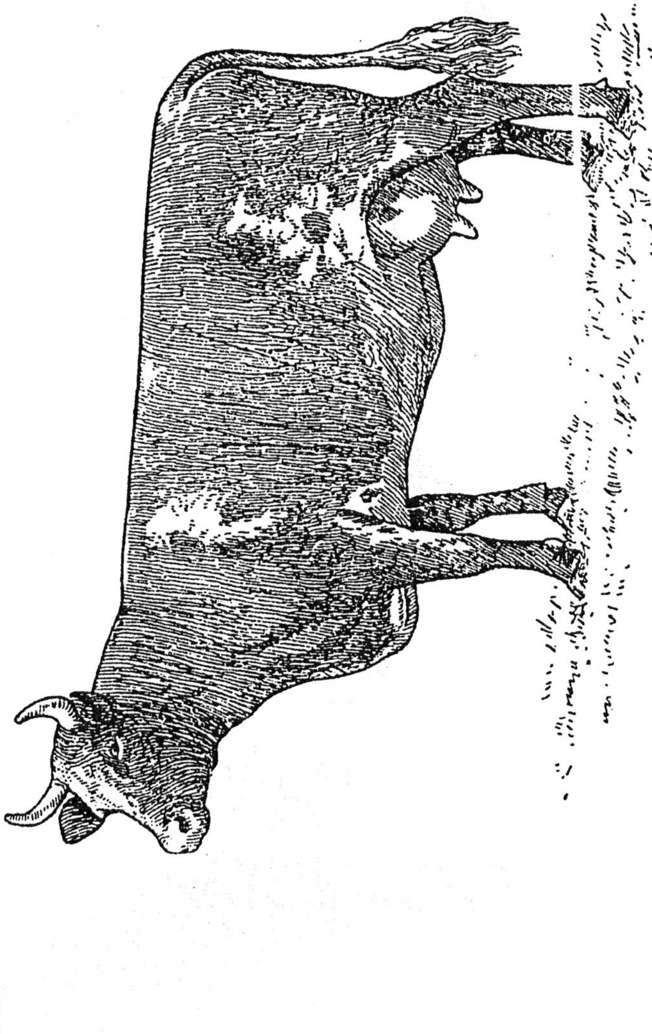

Fig. 32: Short Horn Dairy Cow, Hawthorn VII

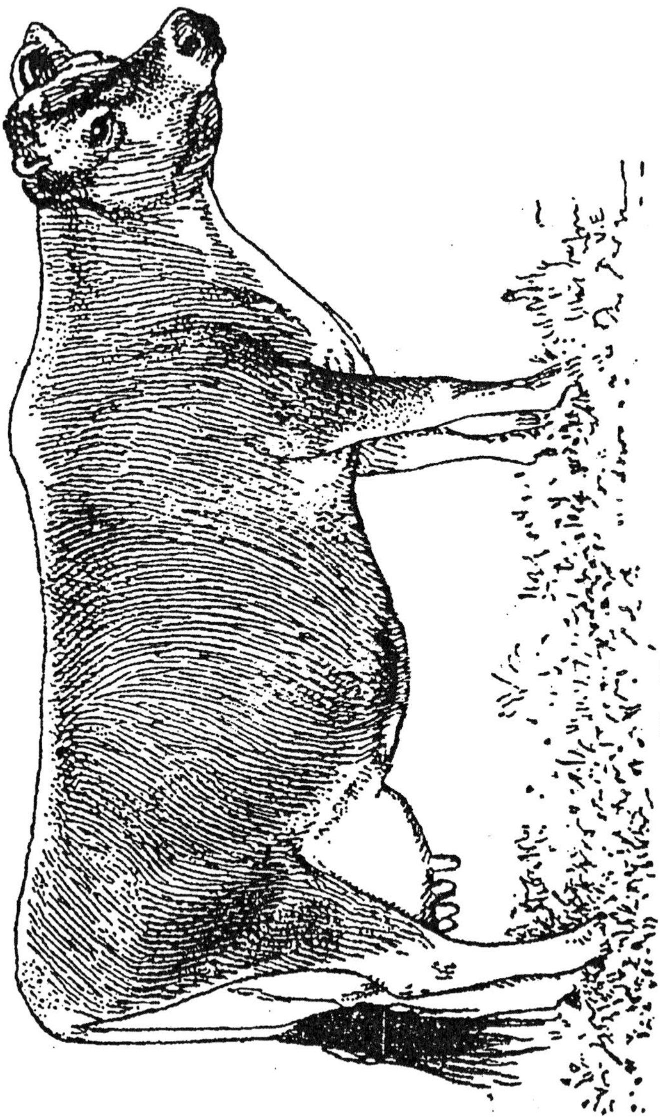

Fig. 33: Jersey Cow, Cute II

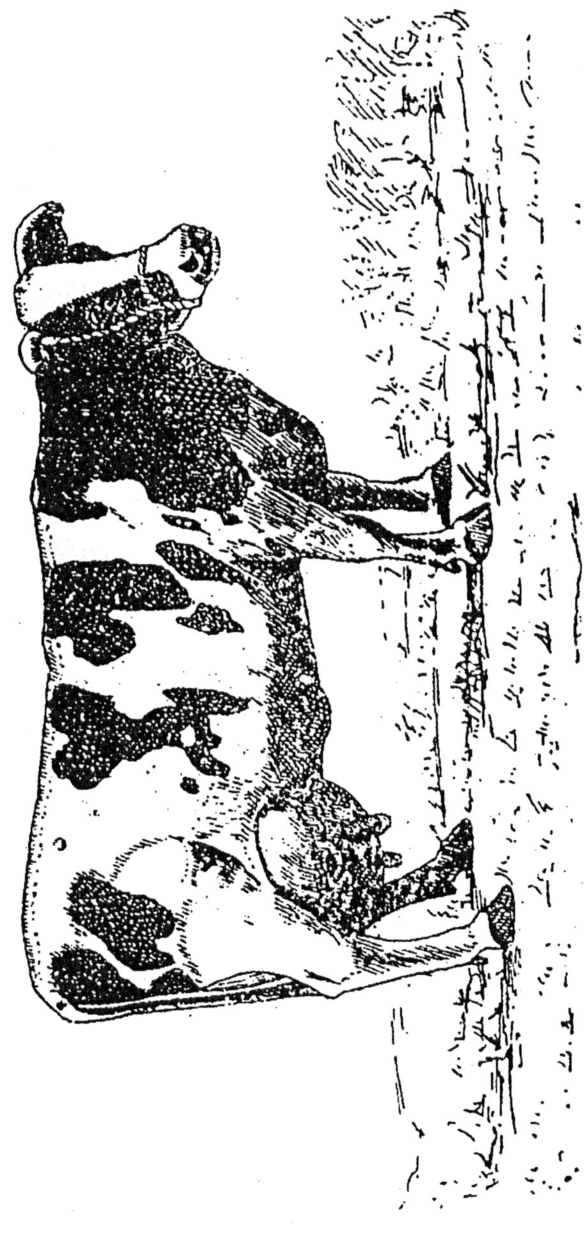

Fig. 34: Holstein Cow, Spotted Daisy Velthuis, Mother of Daisy Grace De Ko.
Seven-day Record: Milk, 578.6 lb., Fat, 18.77 lb., Test, 3.24%, at 10 yrs. 1 mo. 26 days.
Owned by Dan Dimmick & Bro., Ohio

the Punjab. Hissar, Montgomery, and Nellore and other cows have been crossed by Short-horn, Ayrshire, and Jersey bulls. These crosses have produced some good milkers, but in most cases the improvement has not been continued long enough in subsequent crosses and this cross-breeding has been discontinued as a result of failure.

This subject will be more fully treated in another chapter.

The Breed to Get

If a person wishes to keep cows for the use of his own family, he should purchase one, two, or three (or as many as he requires) pure ones, of the Montgomery, Sind, Hissar, Nellore, Mooltan, Gir or Goorgaira breed; or else good cross-breds of the first crossing between the cows of the country and bulls of the above pure breeds. It is always better to buy cows of the district one lives in, if he is in a district that produces good cows, than to import them from another district. If one happens to live in a district where there are no good cows, then he must get them from the nearest district that produces them. No cow giving less than 3,600 pounds of milk in the year is worth the trouble and expense of keeping. Some pure-bred Montgomery, Sind, and Hansi cows will give from 6,000 to 8,000 pounds of milk in one lactation, i.e., from the time they calve to the time they run dry. There are cows (Hansi) that milked for, twelve months, and gave more than 7,000 pounds of milk in that time.

With proper care and feeding there is no reason why the best cattle of the pure Montgomery, Sind, Mooltan, and Goorgaira breeds will not thrive in Bengal and Bihar. They are not very large, and are not very large eaters. They are strong and healthy, and they breed well and their calves thrive nicely. They yield a large quantity of rich milk for a long period and are very profitable; but they will not stand neglect and starvation.

Cross-bred cows between Montgomery bulls and better class Bengali cows have proved good milkers; some of them have given as much as sixteen pounds of milk daily.

Chapter 3

Buying Cows

Quantity of Milk Required

Before buying cows, a person should first consider how much milk he will require daily. He then will know exactly how many cows he needs to buy.

If a cow in full milk gives twenty pounds of milk a day, she should average twelve pounds per day for eight months, and will remain dry for three or four months. A good cow, with proper care, should give a calf every thirteen or fourteen months. Kolkata accordingly one can see how many cows are need to keep him regularly supplied with the required quantity of milk.

If wanted for the use of the family, and if no cow has yet been purchased, the following plan may be adopted. To begin with, buy only one cow in full milk; four months later buy another one, and a third one after another four months. By doing this, a full supply of milk will be secured regularly throughout the year for years. When the first cow is half through her time of milking the second one will come in; by the time the first one stops milking the third one will come in, and by the time the second stops and the third one is half through her time, the first will calve again; and when the third one stops and the first is half through the second will calve again, and so on. But this together with the presupposed proper care and management, otherwise all three cows may stop milking together. This method should be adopted by all good dairymen and farmers. Instead of one cow we can buy as many as we need every four months.

If a very large supply of milk be wanted, and a large number of cows has to be kept, and it is not practicable to keep them when they run dry, then cows in full milk should be bought, and put to the bull after they have milked for three or four months, and when they run dry they should be sold and replaced by others that have newly calved. These cows should if possible be sold to people living in the mofussil, who have grazing ground and can take care of the animals. The purchaser of these cows may be encouraged to revive the good old *Poshani* or *Palani* system which was in vogue in Bengal and is still in existence in some places. In this a person is contracted to keep a heifer of another person and return the same immediately after the 2nd calving-he himself enjoys the milk of the Ist lactation and retains the Ist calf. They should never be sold to butchers or dealers in the city or town. This plan may suit some dairymen whose only object is to make as much money in as short a time as possible, but is not the wisest or best plan for the family and economical dairyman to pursue. For the family, as well as wise dairy farmers, the first plan is the cheapest and safest.

Good cows are not easily procured, and when a person has one, he ought to keep her at all costs. She will amply repay him; besides, it is not only a great pity, but a decided loss to the country, and a crime, to sell good cows to butchers.

If anyone has really good cows that have not been spoiled that they wish to sell, they ought to advertise them. Many European and Indian gentlemen would be only too glad to buy them, and would pay the same prices butchers usually give. This will save the cows from premature slaughter and hence can be utilized for dairy purposes and breeding.

The highest price a butcher will give for a fat cow is Rs. 60. The usual price he pays for dry cows is from Rs. 30 to 40. When people have good dry cows for sale they should advertise them and be willing to sell them to people in the country, who will keep them and breed from them, for the same prices offered by butchers.

Servants' Tricks

Now, the next thing to do before purchasing the cow is not to allow your servants to have a hand in the transaction. All servants, from the sirdar bearer down to the mehter, will conspire to prevent their master from profiting by the possession of cows. The khansama would much rather that milk and butter be bought, as he not only takes a percentage–*dustoori*–on all bills, but also levies a fee upon the milkman for his khansamaship's patronage. The bearer must have his commission from the man who sells the cow to his master, and the man who will give the largest commission is sure to get the preference; and though the cow be an inferior or diseased one, he will pronounce it perfectly good, and persuade his master to buy it, and will prevent other and better cows being brought to his master. Thus, the oftener cows have to be sold and new ones bought, the greater is his gain. The cook also prefers to buy the butter and ghee for the use of the kitchen, and put down six *chittacks* in his account when he has only used four. A careful housekeeper will measure the milk and butter, and thus make herself disagreeable in more ways than one; so, as a rule, all table-servants and cooks set themselves against their masters keeping cows, and if they have a hand in the matter, they will do all they can to make the cows failures. If the bearer or any other servant is allowed a hand in the purchase of the cows, or in their feed and keep, he will be sure to make them at least an expensive luxury.

On account of servants' tricks, it is almost impossible to get any article of food or drink in its original purity. In order to give *dustoori* the sellers are obliged to adulterate the things, otherwise where would be their gain? One reason why gowallas water their milk and otherwise adulterate it is they have to make up for the heavy commissions they have to pay. If a milkman is honest and will not adulterate, his milk, and refuses to pay *dustoori*, he soon finds his milk is condemned and rejected and he loses his customer. The servants can so easily spoil the milk and blame the milkman for giving bad milk, that it is impossible for any milkman to be honest so long as the servants are allowed to meddle with him and the milk.

Indian gentlemen too suffer very much from the dishonesty of their servants. Before a man can sell anything to a raja or zemindar, he has to bribe the servants and hangers-on, from the son-in-law down to the paik or syce. In order to do this the seller has to increase the price of his goods; thus the Indian gentleman has to pay his dishonest relatives and servants for the privilege of buying even a cow or a donkey.

In keeping cows, comfort to the family must be combined with profit to the purse.

Buying a Cow with a Calf

If a cow that has calved be purchased, she should be brought to the buyer's house immediately after calving, and kept under proper treatment until the calf is three weeks old. Bad management at such a time will permanently spoil a cow. A cow is not in full milk until the twenty-first day after calving, and during this period she is liable to many ailments.

Buying a Cow in Calf

If a dry cow be purchased she should be bought at least a fortnight or month before her time for calving, so that she might get used to her new house and attendant. If the cow be one that the intending purchaser knows, or if she be recommended by a trustworthy person who really knows something about cows, then it is well to buy her before she has calved, otherwise the risk of being cheated is great.

There are many advantages in buying dry cows (*see* Chapter 12), but one has to be careful.

If the intending purchaser be not a good judge of cattle, he ought to get the help of some one preferably a Veterinary Surgeon even if he has to pay him for his services.

Selecting a Cow that has Calved the First Time

Although there is an old saying that a cow cannot produce both "milk and beef," says the Australian *Farm Journal*, yet in selecting heifers, we are generally on the look out for what we hope will eventually become a "general purpose" cow. To the man who holds the opinion that "if a cow milks well during her life it matters not what her end is," these remarks will not apply, as the majority of farmers do not hold that opinion. What is required is an animal that will give a good account of herself all through her life, and will finish up something more than a bag of bones; also we require an animal that will breed a good calf, which will pay if kept for rearing, or will readily sell for that purpose. In selecting the animals, perhaps the chief point to obtain is a good consistution, and herein a breeder has a distinct advantage over a buyer who does not know the parentage of the animals he selects. There are certain points which indicate robustness or otherwise.

To judge a young cow correctly, she should be seen a few days, after calving, when her udder is at its best, and shows its capabilities, for as milk is her principal product, the size, shape and milk producing capacity of this is naturally important. It should be large, square, and well set. The teats, which should be moderately long enough to allow full-handed milking, should be set well apart, though it should be remembered that the teats get bigger by using and therefore smaller teats are to be preferred to very large ones in a cow with her first calf. They should be equidistant and set square on the udder, and should be of even thickness; thick or thin-necked teats should be avoided. Whilst lying well forward under the belly, it is of equal importance that the udder should show well behind, filling up between the thighs and extending upwards.

There ought to be plenty of loose skin at the back part; this is an indication of greater possibilities in the future. The milk veins, which run on each side of the belly to supply blood to the udder, should be well developed and not too thin.

General Appearance

First, a young cow should certainly be feminine-looking, rather broad across the eyes and forehead, eyes prominent and mild in expression and temperament. Beware of an animal that is bad tempered and has a very wild, scared look, fine muzzle, and fine tapering horns. Masculine-headed cows are not always to be relied upon as regular breeders, and very rarely give very great satisfaction in the milk-pail. The neck should be fairly long, and should taper from the shoulders, carrying the head level and firm. The shoulders should be well-built and sloping, rather narrower at the top, but with plenty of width below; forelegs well apart, showing an expansive chest. A narrow-chested weak animal should not be kept; she should have well-sprung ribs, and a capacious stomach to hold and digest plenty of food, and supply the other parts of the body with nutriment.

The back should be long and straight, with strong loins, hind legs well set apart, so as to leave plenty of room for the udder, and the skin should be fairly thick, soft, and loose, and should feel mellow to the touch, with fine hair covering it.

Beware of thin, hard skins; they usually denote a bad constitution. The tail should be fairly long and tapering, with plenty of hair at the end. One great point to remember when buying young cows is that if one wishes to purchase good stock he must not expect to find them in the open markets or public sales.

Pay a Good Price

Plenty of patience is required, and one must be prepared to wait some time, and when the opportunity occurs, with careful selection and paying a good price, one is usually able to purchase a good animal for his purpose. This is far better than buying inferior animals at a smaller price, just because they happen to be there and seem cheaper. The difference in produce will soon make up the extra cost, and one will possess a herd of cows suitable for his purpose.

Chapter 4

Points in a Good Cow

Outward Appearance

A good cow is loose-limbed and has a large body; her head is small and her forehead fairly broad; her coat is soft and silky, and her tail thin and flexible, with a rich and glossy (often wavy) bunch of hair at the end; her horns point backward, not forward, though occasionally a good cow with horns pointing forward is met with; she has short legs, wide hips, and a deep and somewhat broad chest, and is long barrelled; her hams are wide apart, as if nature had intended her to have a large udder when in milk. Viewed from the side she should be wedge-shaped. In a heifer the milk-vein is not visible, but when a cow is about to calve, if she is going to be a good milker, it will be very apparent, and will have the appearance of a cord running along the lower part of her stomach; her teats will be well developed and large and set evenly apart.

The limbs of a good cow are loose and large, and the flesh on them rather hangs downwards. A fat, sleek cow is probably a gross feeder, and what she eats runs into fat.

Neatly built heifers, with nicely rounded limbs and a tendency to fat rumps (not hams), usually do not prove to be good cows.

Temper

A good cow is slow and lazy in her movements, and looks motherly. Brisk, frisky cows are seldom good milkers, and very often are vicious and troublesome at milking time. A good milker is of a dull, quiet temperament, and only becomes excited when her calf is frightened or touched by a stranger. Some are so good-tempered that they will allow even strangers to touch them and their calves, without getting in the least excited. A cow with her first calf is more excitable than an older one.

Colour

Black, dark brown, and red cows are generally believed to be healthy and strong. The milk of a red cow is generally supposed to be the sweetest. Red cows, generally, have good digestion, and there is a belief among the people that the milk of a black coloured cow is the sweetest. A greyish white is a very common colour in India; a cow of this colour at some seasons will be quite white, and at others a dark grey. This colour is not confined to any special breed, but as a rule such cows are not bad milkers. When the grey takes the form of piebald, the cow will probably prove a very good one. A creamy white denotes richness of blood, and if at the same time the inside of the ears and the hoofs be a bright yellow, the milk will be very rich and produce a large quantity of butter; and if the hair be also fine, the cow will, in all probability, prove a large milker as well as a rich one.

The milk of a pearly or bluish white cow, with little or no yellow in her skin, often becomes poor and bluish.

Quality of Milk

Every cow gives milk of a different quality and colour. When selecting a cow, the quality and colour (as well as the quantity) of her milk must be taken into consideration. If the cow is in milk, take a little of her milk in a clear wine glass and examine it. If the milk be of a, bluish hue it is poor. There is generally a good deal of *serum* in the milk of cows that are very large milkers, and such milk does not produce much cream or butter, but it is exceedingly good for young children. The yellower the milk the better; therefore a cow giving yellow milk is more valuable than one giving bluish milk. Many cows that give rich yellow milk make up in quality what they lack in quantity. Cows giving a very large quantity of milk are exceedingly delicate, as all their strength runs into milk, and sometimes they leave off calving earlier than they should. A cow that gives from twenty to twenty-four pounds of milk a day is a first-rate one for all practical purposes."–*Cows in India.*"

Milking qualities, as every cow keeper knows, are largely hereditary. The progeny of a heavy-milking cow are likely to inherit the characteristic of their dam. Gallon records are certainly useful in testing the milk-yielding capacity of the cows; but there is the matter in point of quality to consider as well as quantity. The butter-maker would prefer to measure the yield in pounds of butter rather than gallons of milk.

The better class of dairy cows generally yield milk richer in butter-fat than do many other cows. A cow yielding less than one pound of butter per day when in full lactation is no good as a butter producer, however many pounds of milk she may give. In the hands of a milk-seller or cheese-maker she may prove a useful animal, but unless she yields butter to the amount of one pound per day she will not pay well as a butter producer.

Blind Nipples

Some cows of the best milking breeds have this blemish. Blind nipples show tendency to gathering in the udder, which is very troublesome, and often renders a cow quite useless. Cows with blind nipples should be avoided. The four nipples should be of the same length and at equal distances apart.

A cow with a blind nipple that has proved in exceptionally good milker can be kept for breeding calves, but not for dairy purposes. Her price will be reduced by at least 50 per cent.

The Cow's Udder

An udder is a sign of milk to most people. The sight of a large loose-limbed cow, rolling along like a ship in distress, with a big heavy bag swinging from side to side, is, to the majority of casual observers, equivalent to looking at an overflowing pail of milk.

If it is said the sign is not altogether a reliable one then it will astonish most people, but so it is. There are udders and udders, and a big bag does not always denote a big milk record. Frequently a large udder does not even look milky, and it is strange that buyers should be deceived by it.

In many cases the bag appears very fleshy and coarse, sometimes it hangs low, and is more after the shape of a bottle with large coarse teats beneath; and invariably such cows will be poor milkers, with a greater propensity towards beef-production than the exercise of their milking functions.

A Big Bag, more often than not, induces ordinary buyers to pay more than they might otherwise think of doing for a milch cow. Sometimes one may come across an animal with a very large and milky-looking udder of perfect shape. But one will not find many of this type in the open market.

The shape of the perfect udder is rather peculiar, and should be easily recognized. In a cow that has been bred with the development of this organ in view, the udder will be seen to hang perpendicularly behind, extending in a straight line along the stomach, parallel with the back. The front quarters will be well developed.

A "milky" udder has a soft, velvety appearance; the skin is elastic and silky to the touch; the milk-vein will be prominently developed, and well branched; small veins will appear on both sides; and the teats are evenly placed wide apart on both sides of the udder. One of the commonest faults is for the teats to be clustered closely together at the bottom of the udder. Often the udder drops too low, and there is very little development in the fore part.

Distending the udder by "stocking up" is still a common practice when cows are being sold in the public market, and by dealers. It is curious that owners should trouble themselves with this very cruel and most injurious practice, for there must be few buyers who would be deceived by so obvious a fraud into admiring the "big bag" that is so exhibited.

May be some people still imagine that a cow with an enormous, over-stocked udder, and the milk escaping from the teats and falling in a thin stream to the ground, must necessarily be a heavy milker; but the stocking-up process does harm to the cow, and the animal may really be a very poor milker.

Frequently cases of garget and inflammation of the udder are the direct results of this practice.

The teats of some cows are very large, and it has become the rule to give preference to large-teated cows. Many people maintain that it is easier to milk such animals than those with small teats.

Certainly the question of size in teats plays no part at all in determining milk production; providing, of course, the milkers are people who are quite accustomed to large or small teats, as the case may be. Often a cow with very small teats is an exceptionally heavy milker.

Naturally, when buying a cow, one makes a careful examination to assure oneself of the soundness of each quarter of the udder. A blind teat reduces the value of a milch cow considerably. In fact, a cow with this blemish is no good as a dairy cow.

This leads on to the question of buying cows when they are dry. It is risky to purchase a dairy cow that is dry, for an unsound quarter, a blind teat, or almost any defect may, of course, be easily hidden at that time.

Generally, cow-keepers sell three-teated cows after their milking period is completed.

Scarred Cows

Because a cow happens to be scarred about the face, neck, or shoulders, it is no reason that she must be rejected. Quacks fire and brand the cows for some of the simplest ailments, and these scars may be the results of severe treatment of some such disease. But a cow should always be thoroughly examined by a Veterinary Surgeon, to see if she is suffering from any disease.

Age

When buying a cow it is best to select a young one; although an older cow will give more and richer milk. A young cow will always sell well after she has milked for five or six years, while an old cow may soon fail to calve or suddenly stop her milk, and thus become worthless. Again, an old cow is subject to many difficulties in calving from which the younger one is exempt. A cow about to have her second or third calf is a good one to choose, as she has got over the difficulties of her first calving, and will give her full supply of milk.

"It costs more to make milk from old cows than it does from young ones having the same milk-producing capacity. The period of profitable milking does not terminate at the same age with all cows. Some hold out longer than others, but as a rule the best efforts do not reach beyond the eighth year of the cow's age. The quantity of milk given generally keeps up until a cow is ten years old, and sometimes considerably longer; but after a cow has reached her eighth year, her milk is produced at a greater cost of feed, and after that age it costs more to fatten her, while her flesh depreciates in quality."–*American Farmer.*

Number of Calves a Cow Has Had

"The value of a cow depends so much on the number of calves she has had that no reliance can be placed on the statement of sellers on this point and the buyer must trust to his own judgment.

"The best way of judging is by the figure. The hips become more prominent, the belly lower, the skinny parts of the body lengthen and hang, and the udder becomes' more raggy after each calf. A cow carrying her first calf shows her condition but little, but an old one decidedly so; with a little experience it is not difficult to determine about how many times a cow has calved.

"It is impossible to tell how often a cow will calve; some have been known to produce as many as twenty, and some have not given more than five. Eight is the average number; after the eighth calf a cow is supposed to be of no marked value, although she may have two or three more calves."–*Cows in India*.

A Good Milker

If the cow brought for sale be in milk, have her milked in your presence. Even if she be nearly dry, it will be easy to judge by the breadth of the stream or flow whether she is a good milker or not. A broad stream shows a good milker, and a thin, poor stream a scanty milker. When a good milker is milked, the milk will rattle against the vessel with a steady rush, and one who has seen cows milked will easily recognize this, particular sound; when the supply is scanty, the milk passages are crude and small, and the milk cannot flow freely.

A good milker will give all her milk at one or two drawings, but a poor milker will need to have the calf mouth her three or four times before all the milk can be extracted.

A Slinker

If a cow has once slipped her calf, she is very liable to do it again, and it is not safe to buy her when in calf. Slinking very often is hereditary.

If a cow has calved much before her full time it is liable to effect the quantity of her milk.

If the calf has died, the mother's milk will rapidly decrease.

Calves

When purchasing a cow, be particular that the calf is as well-bred as its mother. The calf's breed will affect the mother's supply of milk as well as its own value (*see* Chapter 14).

The Wedge Shape

Judging cows by external appearance, is a difficult matter to dogmatize on, because it is not uncommon to find good milking cows of an ugly shape. At the same time it is admitted that the cow which produces most at the smallest cost does possess what are called dairy characteristics of form. This has been brought out in an experiment to find out the cost of the production. Cows of all breeds differed, but the conclusion on the whole was that the economical cows had the true dairy appearance (wedge shape), while the costly ones had the beef build and appearance.

This is satisfactory, as reconciling theory with practice, but in putting forward dairy characteristics the mistake is sometimes made of overdoing the wedge shape, and thus running the risk of want of constitution. It is apt to be forgotten what a great strain on the system continued deep milking implies, and how essential it is to have a frame strong enough to stand this. We judge constitution by the heart, and we want room up and down and through. We do not want a deep narrow cow, or a shallow broad cow. She must have lots of room for the heart and lungs, because these are the organs upon which the animal must depend for its life.

Chapter 5

Food

Proper Care and Treatment of Milking Cows

Cows are delicate creatures, and their supply of milk greatly depends upon the management and care they receive. Naturally this supply is only sufficient to feed the calf, but under proper care and management it largely exceeds this amount. As a highly cultivated plant when neglected returns to its wild state, so cattle if not properly cared for, will soon deteriorate, and the milk of the cow will greatly diminish and sometimes altogether stop. Proper care and treatment are essential to keep up the unnaturally large supply of milk.

It is very easy to spoil a cow, and if owners do not exercise unremitting vigilance, it will be impossible to keep their cows in full milk and good health, and their bulls and bullocks in working order. In addition to vigilance, they must know something about the treatment of cattle both in health and sickness, when in milk or when dry. These are facts that very few people in India seem to understand.

Food

The cow's food is one of the things that needs the most careful attention. Cows are clean and fastidious feeders, and every cow will not eat the same kind of food. The feeding utensils must be kept perfectly clean and free from any disagreeable smell, or else the cow will not eat her food. If anything offensive have chanced to get into the food, the cow will refuse the whole of it; sometimes it happens that a little piece of dung will get into the straw or *bhoosa*, or in the oilcake, and the whole of the food will be wasted. The water that the food is mixed with must be perfectly clean. Bad food or water will seriously affect the milk.

Fowls, sheep, goats, pigs, and dogs should not be allowed to go near the dairy or cattle food. People suffering from any disease must be kept away from cows and calves.

Some food should always be given to the cow immediately before she is milked, as the rush of milk on an empty stomach tries her strength. A pound of wheat-bran sprinkled over the food that remains in the feeding-trough in the morning is all that is necessary.

In the hot weather after the cow has been milked early in the morning she should be let out to graze until eight or nine o'clock, then she must be brought in and given her regular morning meal. In the cold weather it is better to give the cow her food early in the morning and let her out to graze and exercise at about nine or ten o'clock.

It is hot wise to keep the cow tied up in her stall all through the day and night. If she is not allowed sufficient exercise she will not keep in good health. The cow should be sent out to graze at all seasons (except when it rains heavily) for two or three hours in the morning. When the cow has been given her food she should be tied up and left alone quiet, to eat her food at leisure. She must be given plentiful supply of good drinking water.

She should have her evening food at six o'clock. Sometimes it is best to give the food in three or four meals instead of two. Some cows will waste a great deal of food if much be given at one time, as the food begins to smell sour in a few houRs.

Regularity in feeding and milking must be strictly observed.

The Kinds of Grain that are Good for Cows

Kullie or *woorid* (black dal), barley, wheat, peas, gram, and rahar are the only kinds of grain that should be given to milch cows; all other grains are more or less injurious. Rice is good for sick cattle, but has not much nutriment. Indian corn fattens, but does not increase milk. Indian-corn bran is better. Khassari should never be given to cattle, goats, or sheep. It is very heating and dries up the milk, and is also very indigestible and stunts the growth. It often produces paralysis. Gram and peas should be given to only heavy milkers and weak cows, and then not more than one or two pounds a day to each.

Rahar-pigeon pea-is also good for cows, but not so good as kullie, gram, or peas. It should be ground into meal and steeped.

Bran is one of the principal "offals" obtained in the milking of wheat. Two forms of bran are sold–the "broad" and the "medium." The former consists mainly of the larger flaky particles of the outer coats of the wheat grain, and especially finds favour for feeding horses; the latter, which consists of the finer particles of the same material, constitutes the bulk of the bran made in this country, and is used mainly for dairy cattle.

Bran is particularly rich in lime and phosphates, and it is therefore specially well suited to young growing animals and brood animals of all kinds both before and after parturition. It is a very palatable food, and this fact, coupled with its well-known laxative influence, peculiarly fits it for feeding in association with such concentrated foods as cotton-cake, oilcake, bean-meal, and maize, and with coarse fodders, such as wheat, barley, or paddy-straw.

In experiments conducted by the Edinburgh and East of Scotland College of Agriculture in 1910-11 and 1911-12 with two-year old fattening bullocks, bran proved equal to linseed cake in respect of the quantity and quality of the beef produced, and was slightly the more profitable feeding stuff. In America bran has been extensively used as a partial substitute for oats in feeding heavy horses and has resulted in a very considerable saving in the cost of maintenance. It was found that these two foods might suitably be mixed in equal proportion for young stock.

Sharps and Middlings

Sharps is a wheat offal of a grade intermediate between bran and middlings, and it consists mainly of fine particles of bran with a certain amount of adherent meal.

Middlings represents the innermost layers removed from the wheat grain when making flour, and this offal closely approaches flour in its general character. Sharps contains as a rule slightly more fibre than middlings, but in all other respects the two are very much alike in composition and may conveniently be considered together.

In general character and feeding properties they closely resemble bran, being rather more nutritious than bran, but lacking in some of the special qualities possessed by that feeding stuff. Sharps and middlings are mainly used in the feeding of pigs and poultry.

Quantity of Food

The following should be divided into two or more meals in, twenty-four hours, and is sufficient for a milch cow of ordinary size giving from twenty to twenty-four pounds of milk, but, a very large cow or cows giving a large quantity of milk need a proportionate quantity of food. Small cows giving eight to ten pounds of milk will need only half or even less the quantity.

Kullie- or Maskullie (*woorid*)	4 lb.
Wheat-bran (*bhoosi*)	2 lb.
Kullie, peas or rahar chooni-bran	3 lb.
Mustard oilcake (*khully*)	2 lb.
Cotton-seed (*bunaula*), gram or pea-meal	1 lb.
Chaff (*bhoosa*), wheat, barley or oats chaff	10 lb.
Green grass, chopped fine	30 to 40 lb.
Salt	2 oz.
Sulphur	½ oz.
Total	62 lb. 2½ oz.

Concentrated fodders are given to dairy cows @ ½ lb. per every lb. of milk-yield, to the maximum of 6 seers and the food should be reduced proportionately as the milk decreases.

Food given in excess than what is necessary is never assimilated and generally produces digestive derangement and the animal should be given sufficient leisure to chew the cud.

In place of cotton-seed one pound of ground gram or peas may be given. Not more than two pounds of mustard oilcake should be given to a milch cow during the twenty-four hours. If linseed, *til*-seed, groundnut, or cocoanut oilcake is procurable, four pounds may be given to the cow instead of two pounds of mustard oilcake and the grain be reduced by two pounds. Groundnut cake is also good for cattle. When green grass cannot be procured, give extra chaff or paddy-straw. Green grass is very essential to health, but during part of the year it is very difficult to get any. In the place of grass give extra chaff, hay, or paddy-straw; give as much as the cow will eat, but it should not be given dry.

The water in which rice has been washed, and the rice-*kanji* or *marh*, are very good for cows and should either be mixed with the food or given separately with little salt or treacle.

The quality of the food must be the best; it is no economy to feed cows upon damaged weevil-eaten grain and bran, or rotten oilcake and straw.

Effects of the Different Kinds of Food

Of the different kinds of grain mentioned above as being the only ones that should be given to cows, kullie (*wood*), also known as maskullie, is the best for milch cows, as it produces milk as well as nourishes. There are two kinds of kullie: one is black and the other is greenish grey in colour. Both are good, but the lighter one is the better. Kullie, wheat, peas, and gram increase the quantity and improve the quality of milk, and strengthen the cow. But in the winter it is best to reduce the kullie and increase the bran, peas, and gram as kullie is cooling, and some cows suffer a great deal from cold. This is given boiled or steeped in water. Gram is the best for calves, bulls and bullocks. Kullie should not be given to calves, bullocks or bulls, nor to dry cows.

If the cow is not strong and is out of condition, the quantity of gram should be increased. Gram is very nourishing.

Wheat-bran is very necessary for cows in calf and for young calves.

Wheat-bran like all other starchy food produces heat and energy and is believed to improve the quality (butter-fat) of milk.

If the cow's digestion is not good, the grain and oil-cake should be decreased and the wheat-bran increased.

If she is a small eater, the chaff and straw should be lessened, otherwise she will waste much of her food.

Green grass gives colour and on account of the vitamin it contains, gives richness to the milk and butter, and keeps the cow in health.

Cotton-seed produces rich butter, but more than one pound a day should never be given to any cow, as it is very heating and difficult to digest, and often causes inflammation of the udder. Some prefer ground gram and peas to cotton-seed. Gram and peas also enrich the milk.

Salt and sulphur are purifiers, they help digestion and keep the bowels in proper condition, acting as preventives against many diseases.

There is not much nourishment in paddy-straw; wheat, barley, and oats straw (*bhoosa*) are much better.

Oilcake helps to produce milk and butter. All oilcakes are not good for milch cows or young calves. The best are those made from *til*, *ulsee*, or *teesi* (linseed), cocoanut and the groundnut. Other kinds of oilcake, *e.g.*, mustard, is a good appetizer and also helps digestion but is very heating and therefore injurious to cows. Linseed and *til*-seed oilcake are good for calves, especially when under three months of age. Mustard-seed oilcake may be given to calves only after they are three or four months old and then only in small quantities to begin with. The oilcake made from the mustard or rape-seed is good for bullocks and bulls and large-growing calves.

The *til* khully is sweet in flavour; it has an oily smell, and is of a chocolate colour, and if old is hard and dry. This is certainly the best for cows, but is rather difficult to procure; even if it costs more than the other kinds, it should be used in preference to any other. Next to the *til* and *teesi* in point of excellence is the cocoanut oilcake. Cows generally do not like it at first, and it should be given fresh and in small quantities until they become accustomed to it. The mustard oilcake is the most common, and generally used; but is not suitable for milch cows and should never be given to calves under three months of age.

All these oilcakes form good nourishing food, and are invaluable for the formation of the various tissues that enter into the formation of the animal structure, to enrich the blood and promote secretion of milk. Great care should be taken that the oilcake is fresh and has no worms or mould in it. The *til* oilcake, especially, soon goes bad and gets full of worms.

Much of the cake produced by oil-mills are unsuited for cattle. Very often chemicals are used to extract all the oil, and these chemicals are highly injurious to cattle.

Preparation of Food

All the grain should always be ground fine and steeped in clean water. Four pints of water should be added to every pound of grain, and then it should be allowed to soak for 3 or 4 hours before feeding, and if allowed to soak longer it ferments and brings in stomach trouble. Kullie should be boiled; or should be ground fine and soaked for hours. When *kullie* is boiled, it seems to disagree with cattle at first, but they soon become accustomed to it.

The wheat-bran should be given dry mixed with the other food, but if the bran be old or there be insects in it boiling water must be poured over it before it is given to cattle or horses.

The cotton-seed should be thoroughly ground, and soaked until it gets quite soft.

The oilcake should be broken up into small pieces, and soaked for 3 to 4 hours.

The chaff, grass, hay, and straw should be chopped into pieces two inches in length.

The salt and sulphur should be ground and added to the grain when put to steep.

All the ingredients should be well mixed with a sufficient quantity of water or rice-*kanji* to make it sloppy.

Great care must be taken that none of the grain is given whole and unsoaked, and that the food is not given dry. The milch cows, during summer specially, should be given a draught consisting of *goorh* (molasses) 1 seer, *satoo* ½ seer and water about 2 gallons, occasionally during mid-day.

Newly calved cows may be allowed daily for 3 to 4 weeks or more in order to incite the full supply of milk.

N.B.–Cows giving milk should never be allowed to grow very fat. When the food goes into fat the milk will decrease, and the cow become barren. In such cases the oilcake and gram should be reduced and the cotton-seed stopped. But the cow must always be kept in good condition.

Cost of Food

The cost of food varies in different parts of the country, and at different seasons of the year, but the food should never cost more than from a fourth to two-thirds the value of the milk the cow gives.

Green Food

Cows should never be deprived of green food; if they are, they will not keep in good health besides, the milk will decrease in quantity and be poor in quality, because green food contains lot of vitamin.

Doob is the best grass for cattle. Young wheat, barley, kullie, peas, Indian-corn stalks, jowar, bajra, and paddy, in their green and tender state, and green tender leaves of fruit trees, are excellent for cattle. The long juicy grass that grows among the Indian-corn, wheat, and other crops makes splendid cattle fodder. Carrots and beetroot chopped up, and, occasionally cabbages, are very wholesome and good food.

Three and a half biggahs or one acre of land is what one cow needs to keep her supplied with green food throughout the year.

The villagers never think of giving their cattle any special food. The poor animals are let loose in the morning and tied up in the evening, and all the food they are allowed is what they manage to pick up in grazing, with the addition of perhaps a handful of dry paddy-straw at night.

Jowar (Sorghum) in its green tender state is splendid food for cattle, but the greatest care must be taken about the condition of the plant, for at a certain stage it is poisonous. The stock and leaves of the jowar and Indian-corn must be cut into pieces one inch in length.

Sorghum Poisoning

In view of the number of cases of sorghum poisoning which occur in India, the following note, taken from the *Queensland Agricultural Journal*, may be of interest:

"A very important discovery with regard to sorghum poisoning was made by Dr. S. Avery, Chemist of the Nebraska Agricultural Experiment Station, who has shown that carbohydrates (sugars, as glucose, milk, sugar and molasses) act as an antidote against the poisonous action of prussic acid and the prussic acid yielding glucoside. The presence of sugars in the first place retards the action of the enzyme in liberating free prussic acid; and, again, prussic acid unites with sugars to form less poisonous addition products. Dr. Avery recommends, therefore, to give to an animal suffering from sorghum poisoning, in a case that its condition still allows medical treatment, a strong solution of glucose syrup or molasses; or, again, a large quantity of milk. Actual experiments have shown that an animal could be given a large dose of pure prussic acid, up to three times the fatal dose, if glucose was given at the same time; the animal became very sick, but still recovered. Farmers have, therefore, a fairly safe remedy in molasses for these cases of poisoning. Treacle is a cheap and valuable cattle food in almost any country, especially for sweetening *bhoosa*, chaff and such like fodders."

Straw

Especial care should be exercised in the selection of the straw given to the cow. Wheat and barley straw are certainly the best that can be given to cattle. Wheat and barley straw are broken up and sold as *bhoosa* chaff. See that it is clean and sweet. Frequently it will be found full of mud, dung, leaves, and thorns, or be musty and rotten.

Paddy-straw has less nourishment, but in Bengal it is the chief article of food for cattle. In selecting paddy-straw, be careful that it is not of paddy grown in swamps or low lands. Insects and fungi attack such straw. Such straw will make the cow sick. The straw of the finer quality of paddy grown on high lands is more suitable. Such straw will be nice and clean, of a light yellow colour, and will smell sweet and clean, and unlike the straw from swampy and low lands will not have saltish taste.

Hay

Cattle are not particularly fond of hay, but they will get used to it. Good, sweet, soft hay may be given in small quantities.

Bhoosa

The leaves and stock of peas, kullie, beans, gram, mussoor, and mung, after the grain has been threshed, is very good for cattle. The *bhoosa* should be broken or cut up into small pieces and mixed with the other food. Care must be taken that the *bhoosa* is clean and sweet.

Well-fed and properly cared-for cows will not eat anything filthy, and can be sent out to graze and exercise without the least fear of their picking up anything harmful to themselves or to their milk.

Salt

If a cow does not get sufficient salt and a little sulphur in her food, she will pick up dry bones or lick earth. Salt helps digestion and keeps her in health.

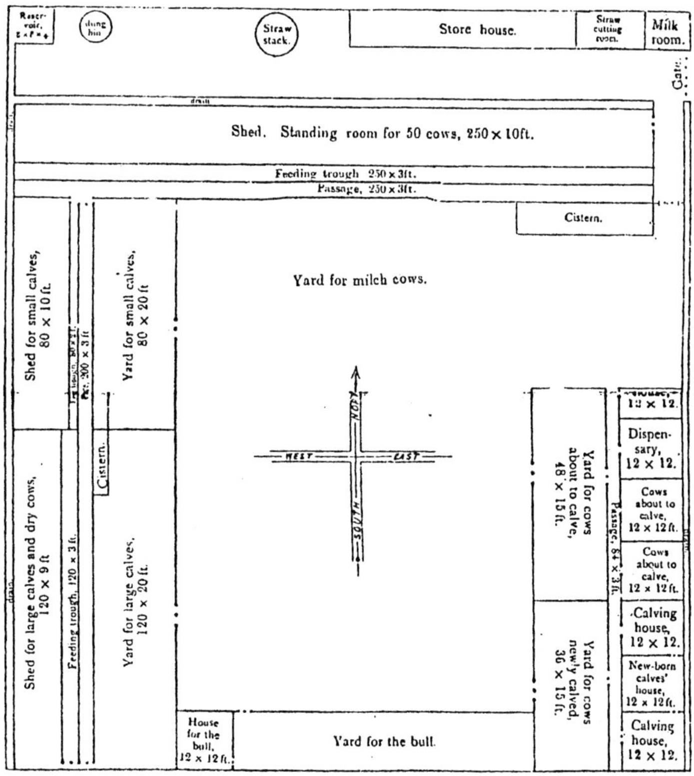

Fig. 35: Model Indian Dairy

Drink

The cow's drinking-water must also be attended to. Pure water and a good supply of it is as absolutely necessary as good and sufficient food. Cows are very thirsty creatures, and if they do not get pure water, at least four times a day, they will drink whatever comes in their way.

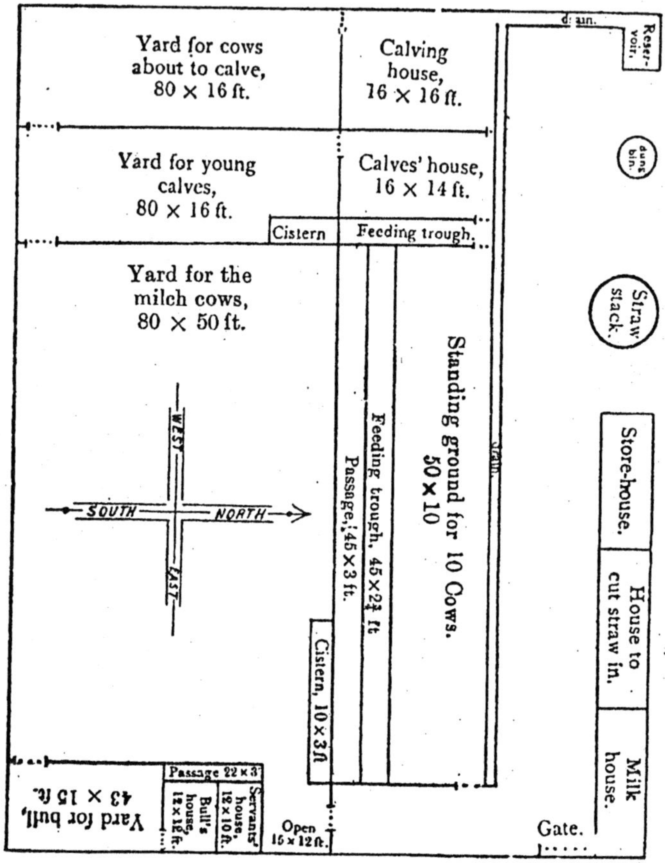

Fig. 36: Model Dairy

Silage

Sour silage should be fed to dairy cattle with caution, for it affects the taste and quality of the milk produced by cows fed on it. If the silage is good and sweet it can be given to milch cows mixed with other food. It can be fed to large calves, dry cows, bulls and bullocks with good results.

Chapter 6

House and Utensils

The cow-house is a very important consideration. Cattle must be properly housed at nights, and sheltered from the midday sun, and from rain and storms.

In the cold weather their house must be free from draughts. In the rains it must be kept perfectly dry. In the hot weather it must be kept open and cool, and at all seasons it must be thoroughly ventilated and cleaned.

It is not at all difficult to build a suitable house for cattle in India. A *pucca* house is preferable to a *kutcha* one, but a very nice one can be built of wooden posts or mud pillars and thatched roof, at a very small cost. Be the house *kutcha* or *pucca*, the floor should ordinarily be of brick and cement. Mud floors are good and convenient for cows but soon wear into holes and become very insanitary and offensive, unless they are dressed properly once or twice a week. Floors made of planks are very dangerous, as cattle slip on them, and are sometimes seriously injured. The best way to make the floor is to put down a lot of broken bricks (*khoa*) and lime, and beat down well; then over this put first-class bricks on edge, well pointed with cement. This flooring will last for years. A cement or patent stone floor is too slippery for cattle.

The level of the floor should be a foot and a half to two feet higher than the surrounding ground.

There are of course many ways of making cow-house. If only one or two cows are kept, a room or two in the out-houses may be appropriated for them, or a stall or two in the stables be given up for their accommodation, but if many cows be kept, a regular cow-house must be built. Whatever the number of the cows, particular attention must be paid to the floor and ventilation.

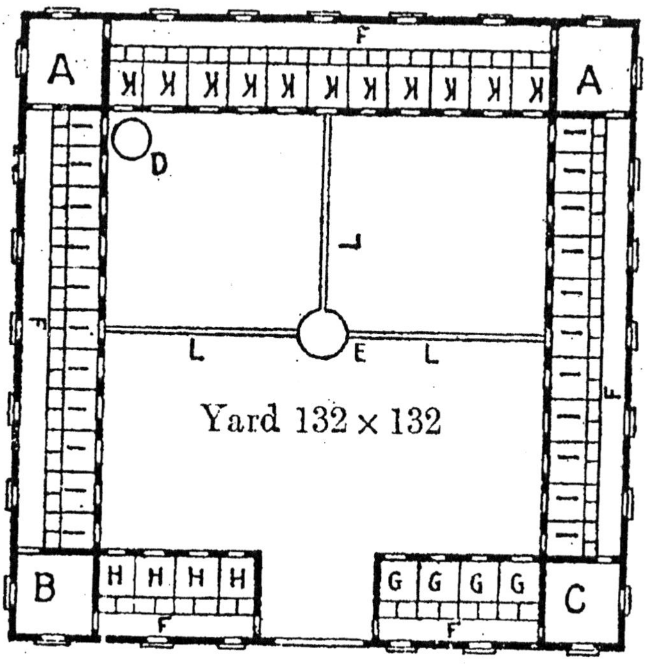

Fig. 37: Model English Dairy

A, store rooms; B, food-preparing room; C, milk room; D, water cistern; E, reservoir; F, feeding passages; G, stalls for calves; H, stalls for calving and newly calved cows; I, stalls for milch cows; K, stalls for dry cows and bull; L, drains.

This is a very simple construction, and can be made as small or as large as necessary. It is divided into three compartments or rooms: one for the cows to calve in, one for the calves when away from their mothers, and one for the larger cattle. The house or houses should always open to the south. The north side must be walled up and have small windows (about 3 feet by 2 feet) 4 feet above the ground and 6 feet apart. The width of the house inside should be at least 6 feet. From the north wall there should be 10 feet of standing ground then 3 feet occupied by the feeding trough, and, lastly, 3 feet for a passage the other side of the trough. The feeding trough to be made of brick and cement running the whole length of the room. The inside of the trough should be from 18 to 21 inches wide, and 12 to 15 inches deep, but the bottom should be raised at least 12 inches from the level of the floor, making it in all 24 inches high. The floor of the house should slope off from south to north-that is, from the head of the cow to her hindquarters. The slope should not exceed 3 inches-just sufficient to carry off all the urine. Right against the north wall there should be a drain to receive and carry off all the droppings. This drain should be 9 inches wide, and 3 inches deep, made of bricks and cement. Outside the cow-house 12 feet from it to the north there should be a reservoir, 4 feet by 4 feet and 2 feet deep, to receive all the urine and water, and the drain of the cow-house should connect with this reservoir.

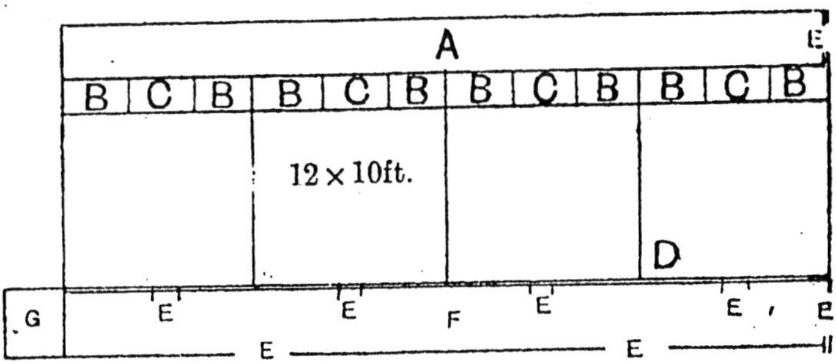

Fig. 38: Stalls for cows, two in each stall. A, passage; B, feeding trough; C, water trough; D, calves' room; E, doors; F, verandah to prepare food; G, reservoir; H, drain.

The roof on the south should be supported by pillars made of either brick, mud or wood. If made of bricks, each pillar should be 24 inches by 15 inches; if of mud, it should be 36 inches by 18 inches; and the opening or doorway between each pillar should not be less than 6 feet wide.

The calving or calves' rooms or houses should be the same as the cows' house; only, for the calves, the feeding trough should be not more than a foot wide, and 6 to 9 inches deep inside; the whole of the trough should not be more than 17 inches high.

Ventilation in this house will be perfect, and it will not be at all difficult to keep the floor perfectly clean and dry at all seasons. During the hot weather, the doors and windows should be kept entirely open during the day and at night; in the cold weather and in rain-storms, the north windows should be kept closed day and night, but the doors should be open during the day and closed only when the nights are very cold. The top part of the doors should have ventilators large enough to admit of sufficient ventilation when the doors are closed.

The doors and windows can be made of mats or wood; the latter is preferable. Purdahs of good stout canvas or tarpaulin also answer well, but are not as good as wooden doors.

The height of the house or room should not be less than 10 feet from floor to ceiling; the doorways should be 8 feet high. If the house be thatched or tiled, the sides should be at least 10 feet, and the centre 15 feet high.

Space

Cattle should never be crowded together. Ample room should be given them to not only stand, but also to sit and lie down comfortably. No cow will keep in good health unless she has 50 feet of standing ground–10 feet by 5 feet. If the cows be large ones, it will be well to allow them each 80 feet of ground-10 feet by 8 feet. For a single cow a room at least 10 feet by 10 feet is necessary, giving her sufficient room to comfortably turn round.

Keeping the floor clean and dry is an indispensable necessity. It must not only be swept clean every morning and evening, but must be thoroughly scrubbed and washed every morning, and swept every time it is soiled. The droppings must not be allowed to remain on the floor or in the drain any length of time. The house must be kept clean and sweet and perfectly dry. Phenyle and water or lime or ash or carbolic powder should be sprinkled on the floor every day. Throwing sand on the floor, or putting down some straw, will prevent cattle from slipping on the *pucca* floor. The cows should be allowed some dry straw to lie on in the cold weather and rains. Especial attention lie on the cold weather and rains. Especial attention must be given to the calves' house and the calving house.

The best time to wash the house is when the cows are let out into the yard in the morning.

Drains

In big cities the drain of the cow-house should, if possible, be connected with the public under-ground street sewer, or else with the reservoir behind the house; already spoken of. This reservoir must be emptied and washed every day, and the contents removed far from the cow-house, and spread over the fields or thrown into the manure pit. The dung should be gathered and kept in a bin at the back of the cow-shed until it is removed in the morning to the manure pit.

Utensils

If only one or two cows be kept, zinc, galvanized or wooden tubs can be used for them. They should be kept perfectly clean, by being thoroughly scrubbed and washed every morning and evening. If these tubs cannot be got, then earthen *gumlahs* (nands) should be fixed on the ground as the people of India do in most villages, but great care is needed to prevent them from smelling offensive, and they should be frequently changed by new ones.

If a number of cattle be kept, the *pucca* cemented trough is the best to have. It will be a great saving in labour. It will take a man nearly half a day to clean a dozen tubs, whereas the trough for the same number of cows can be properly cleaned in half an hour. Besides cattle eat with more comfort out of a raised trough than they do out of tubs.

When milch cows and dry cows and bullocks are kept in the same house, the trough should be divided into two or three divisions, for the same food will not be given to all. If possible, dry cows should be kept in separate rooms or houses from milch cows. Bullocks and bulls may be kept in one house.

The tubs and troughs must be thoroughly scrubbed and washed every morning and evening.

Cistern

There should always be a cistern in every cow-house. The best position for it is immediately outside of the shed on the south in the yard (see sketch of cow-house). This cistern should always be kept filled with pure drinking-water. It should be properly cleaned and refilled every morning. When the cows are let out into the yard, they can have a good refreshing drink. Cattle should be watered at least four times a day.

Mode of Tying

If only one or two cows be kept, they should be tied to separate pegs far apart, that they may not reach each other; but when a number are feeding at the trough, they must be so tied that they will not reach one another. The best mode of tying them is this, put down thick iron rods as posts 5 feet apart all along the trough; to these posts tie good stout pieces of rope or chain.

Each rope is 7 feet long, and is tied by the two ends to two posts, one on either side; to the centre of this rope another rope about 4 feet long is attached, which goes round the cow's neck, and so secures her that she cannot reach her neighbour to the right or left, but at the same time she has ample freedom to stand erect and to sit or lie down with comfort. The ropes should be tied to the top of the posts on a level with the top of the trough. A better plan would be to have iron rings round the posts, and tie the ropes to the rings. This would enable the animal to sit or rise with greater ease, as the ring will slide up or down the post as necessary. Chains can be kept cleaner than ropes.

Bullocks and large calves should be tied in the same manner as the cows, but bulls must be tied far apart with very strong ropes or chains, as they will do much damage if they happen to break loose.

The Yard

When it is not possible to allow the cows to go out into the fields to graze, the cow-house should have a yard attached to it, in which milch cows can be let loose for a couple of hours in the morning and evening. This freedom and exercise are very necessary, and will be very beneficial to the animal's health. The yard should be in front of the cow-house. Each animal should have at least 1,000 feet of ground-50 feet by 20 feet-in the yard, but the more given the better. Dry cows, bullocks, and calves should be sent to graze or kept loose in the yard during the day after their morning meal.

Other Houses

The servants' houses and the store house should be detached

from the cow-house, at least 50 feet from it, or else on the west of the house in the same line. There should also be a little room for keeping the milk utensils and receiving and measuring the milk. If possible, the bull's house should be detached from the main building, and should have a separate yard (as in Figs. 35 and 36).

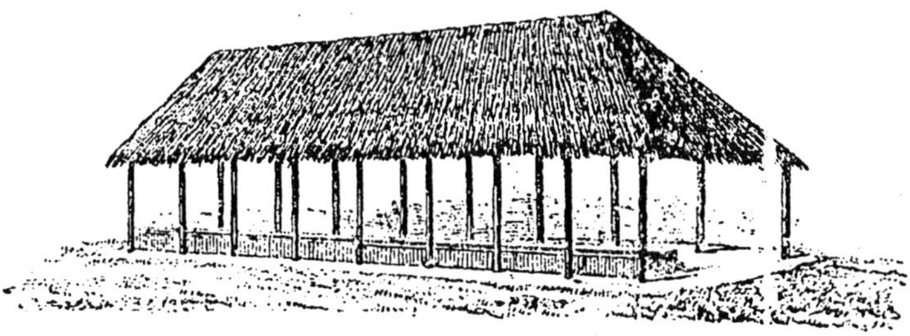

Fig. 39: Cow-shed

A good study of the ground plan of the cow-sheds herein given, will clearly show the reader what is necessary in such an establishment.

Chapter 7

Attendants

In order to keep cows with any degree of success, it is necessary to have proper servants. A great many people buy cows and engage gowallas, and have the poor animals to the tender mercies of these men, and are exceedingly surprised when they find in a few months that the cows are spoiled, or the calves have died. Others, again, put the cows in the care of the bearer or khansama, and cannot understand why the animals give so little milk, or why their food costs so much. So they conclude that keeping cows is a failure, and that Indian cows do not give much milk, and the calves never live. People must always remember that there is a right and a wrong way of doing a thing, and if a person goes the wrong way about it, he must expect failure. If one desires to derive any pleasure and profit from keeping cows, he must attend to them himself, having them under his immediate supervision. If the servants or any other person be entrusted with their management, the enterprise will end in failure and disappointment.

While one personally looks after the animals, he will need servants to do the work and carry out his instructions.

If only one cow be kept, the syce's wife or the wife of some other servant can well look after her, if she is paid two to four rupees a month. But if two or more cows be kept, it will be necessary to have servants specially for them. One man cannot take care of more than six cows, but it is best for him to have only two if in milk; if more be given him, they will not be properly cared for, especially if he has also to milk them and care for the calves.

The Servant's Disposition of Mind

The temper of the cowman has a great deal to do with the health and temper of the animals under his care. He must not only be clean and active, but must also have a love, or at least a liking, for the cows, and be kind and gentle to them. If he is harsh and rough, and drives them about they will become excited and cross, will not eat their food properly, and will give trouble at milking. Cattle get thin and sickly under harsh treatment. A bad-tempered servant should never be kept under any consideration.

Servant's Fidelity

Then, again, the cowman must be faithful, and not only an eye-server. True, such a man among servants would be difficult to get, but the servants must be taught to be faithful to the animals under their care; otherwise, when the master and mistress happen to be away from home, or sick for a day or two, the cattle will suffer. It need never be expected that the servants will give the animals the same care and attention as the master or mistress will give, but they can be made to understand what is expected of them, and that they must do the work properly if they want to serve. It takes a long time, sometimes, months, to get this idea properly instilled into their minds. If the servants see that the master and mistress are careful and watchful, it will make them more attentive.

Most of the servants imagine they know more about cattle than their masters do. In some cases, it is true, owners of cattle are more ignorant than their stupid servants. The prejudice and ignorance of them are hard to overcome. They are unwilling to do anything their grandfathers and great-grandfathers did not do. The custom of their part of the country is law with them.

Chapter 8

Washing, Grooming and Exercise

Washing

Cattle should be kept perfectly clean. When in health they should be regularly washed, bathed once or twice a week or sometimes daily in the hot-weather, once or twice a week in the rains, and once or twice in a month in the cold season. A small quantity of phenyle or Jayes fluid may be added to the bath water. A bright sunny day should be selected for washing. The animals must be thoroughly dried and let loose after the bath. Great care must be taken to prevent them from taking a chill. Milch cows are very liable to chills. Suckling calves should preferably not be bathed.

Special attention should be paid to their feet. See that there is no dirt or stone or thorn between their hoofs and no sore. Wash the feet and clean the hoofs everyday with phenyle and water. If their feet are not attended to, worms may form in sores and the cow be seriously injured.

Grooming

Cattle should be properly groomed every day. The same kind of brush as is used for the horse or gloves made up of cocoanut ropes should be used for the cow. Proper and regular grooming will keep the cattle in good condition, and will prevent their having lice and ticks. Little calves ought to be brushed and the ticks, etc., picked off every second day or so.

Exercise

Cows need regular exercise; working bullocks have enough of it, but milch cows and calves should be let out to graze and exercise for a few hours every day. It is a great mistake to keep them tied up all the time. Close confinement causes disease.

Dry cows, heifers, and large calves should be let out to graze the whole day. A bull needs lots of exercise too; he should be tied up with a long stout rope-40 feet long-in the yard, or if there be an enclosed yard, let loose in it. In advanced stage of pregnancy, cows should not be allowed out with other cattle. She should be tied out with a long rope in the yard or field, and not allowed to run, jump, or fight.

Protection

Cattle need protection from the midday sun and heavy rains. If there are no large trees on the grounds, under the shade of which the cattle can stand, then they should be taken into the shed during the hottest hours of the day, and when it rains heavily, or when the winds are cold and damp. If they are exposed to the hot sun, heavy rains and cold nights they will never keep well. Calves especially are very susceptible to cold and damp, and many are killed by exposure and neglect. During cold weather nights they need to be kept in a warm pen, room or box with sufficient ventilation.

Chapter 9

Breeding

Breeding one's own cows is the surest method of attaining success in the dairy and farm. When a cow is bought one is not at all sure of her blood; she herself may be a large and rich milker, and may milk for a long time, but one is not sure of her producing the same qualities in her progeny. Her parents may not have been of a good milking strain, and though she herself is a good cow, her calves may not be half so good. It sometimes happen that inferior mothers produce very superior slaughters, but this does not occur very often. The general rule is that like produces like. An inferior or unhealthy cow should never be bred from. It is not desirable to breed from a cow whose grandparents as well as mother and father were not as superior as herself. Very often cows as well as other animals throw back-that is, the young ones do not take after the mother and father but after the grandparents. Breeding one's own cows is very often cheaper than buying them. If one has sufficient grass-lands, he will find it more economical to breed than to buy. But it will not pay in cities, where it is impossible to have sufficient ground for the cows to exercise and keep in health, and where one has to pay heavily for every morsel the cows cat. Then, again, in breeding one's own cattle one avoids contagion. Disease is often brought into a dairy through cows that have been purchased.

It is Cheaper to Breed One's Own Cows

The calf has to be kept ten months, or as long as the cow gives milk. If properly cared for and managed, the heifer will take the bull when she is two years or two years and three months old, and yield her first calf by the time she is three years old. So one has to keep the animal for two years and two months after her mother stops milking and before she has her first calf. The cost of her keep and food for these twenty-six months will not exceed from Rs. 80 to Rs. 100. This is less than half the value of a really good cow. If the heifer, when she calves, gives eighteen to twenty pounds of milk a day, she will sell for at least Rs. 250-just double what she bas cost for food and keep.

The art of breeding is governed by a few rules which are simple and easy to understand; and these rules must be faithfully observed if any degree of success is to be gained.

The first and most important of these is that "like produces like," by which is meant that animals of certain peculiarities of form, colour, disposition, habit, health, and quality, when carefully selected and bred together for some generations, as a rule, reproduce their own characteristics in their progeny. This rule has been so uniformly and constantly proved by practice, and is so reasonable and natural, that it may be taken as a safe guide in rearing cows. Every person may see it proved by practice every day of his life. There is more or less of family likeness in the lower animals as well as in human beings. The calf of a Hansi cow and Hansi bull is always a Hansi, and the same is true of all other breeds. Parents of rich milking strains produce a large percentage of calves that will be good milkers, and bear a close resemblance to themselves in all valuable points.

Generally cow-calves take after their fathers, and in breeding the greatest care is needed in the selection of the stud-bull. The bull should always be superior to the cow, and must be of a good milking strain. Both the bull and cow should be the best specimen of their breed (*see* Chapter 10).

1st. Never use an inferior bull. The greatest care must be taken in the selection of the bull.

2nd. Never breed from an inferior cow. Only the best cows must be bred from.

3rd. To improve the breed, the cow must be served by a bull that is superior to her. If the bull be inferior to the cow, the calf will be inferior to the mother; but if the bull be superior to the cow, the calf will be superior to the mother.

4th. Be careful about in-breeding, that is breeding from father and daughter, son and mother, brother and sister. When breeding from close relations the progeny usually deteriorate, unless the greatest care is exercised in selecting only those who are absolutely free from disease and serious defects, and are perfectly healthy and strong and have the good characteristics of the breed in a very marked degree. Line-breeding-that is, breeding in line from selected individuals of the same breed and strain but of different families-should be practised.

5th. Breed from thoroughbred individuals of the same breed. If it is necessary to put the cow to a bull of another breed, he should be of a better breed than the cow. The best breeds to breed from are the Montgomery, Sind, Hissar, and Ongole.

6th. To breed successfully, proper food and careful management are necessary.

An experienced dairyman and large breeder writes thus:

"The calves are the means for the improvement of the dairy. By a gradual course of breeding, rearing, and development, the calves become the basis for all the skill of the dairyman's work in improving his stock, and in increasing their valuable product. Breed is made up of food and the most skilful care; and by judicious management the calves are developed into more useful and productive animals than their dams, until in course of time the improvement becomes fixed, and is inherited by the progeny. It is in this way that the improved breeds have been made up".

"The feeding of a heifer should be liberal. She should have regular rations of the food prepared and given to cows, and about half as much of it will be eaten profitably. Liberal feeding of good food develops the digestive functions, and the training of a heifer for the dairy should be such as to encourage the healthful disposal of as much food as possible. It does not matter if the heifer should get fact, if the growth is not stunted by it. The gradual development of the normal figure of the model cow should be watched, and as long as this development is going on satisfactorily the feeding may be persevered in. Excessive fatness, however, is a bar to usefulness in the dairy, and when heifers with this tendency to fat come in, there is usually some defect which spoils the animals for a dairy cow".

"Breed is undoubtedly dependent upon food as well as upon proper selection of the breeding stock. Feeding and training have given the value to the breed, and this value must be kept up by feeding and training. The mistake is often made of getting a pure-bred animal, and subjecting it to all the careless management which is given to the common stock, and expecting that this animal, by virtue of its parents' character, can lift up the common herd and double or treble its value in a few years. Such a hope is doomed to disappointment from the outset. When a pure animal is brought into a herd, its care should be at least equal to that which it has been used to, and the very same system of feeding and general management should be followed with the whole herd. If this practice is followed success will be sure, and the desired end will be reached."

"The training of heifers for their duties in the dairy should be a constant, care of the dairyman. Vicious animals, which kick, hold up their milk, suck themselves and practice the other usual vices of disorderly cows, are all made so by want of, or misdirected training. The first lesson the calf learns should be affection for its owner, fearlessness and docility. Having never been maltreated it has no sense of fear, and accepts the attention of its owner without alarm. Receiving nothing but kindness and its food from him, it is always ready to meet him with eagerness, and soon learns to come at his call. Its natural instincts are even readily controllable, because its acquired docility accustoms it to give way to the management of its owner, and it never practices those vices which are intolerable in a dairy. It becomes in every respect a domesticated animal; and to attain this result, with all the comfort and advantages it involves, should be the constant care of the dairyman whose crop of calves is being harvested. Kindliness and gentleness in the owner are indispensable to these virtues in his cattle."–*H. Stewart*.

More will be said upon this head in the chapter upon Calves and their Management.

The Dual Purpose Cow for India

By W.M. Smith

Assistant Director, Dairy Farms, Southern Circle

In most European Countries and America an attempt has been made at some time or other to evolve by breeding and selection what is known as the dual purpose cow, which in the case of the countries above mentioned means a cow capable of fulfilling two distinct and diametrically opposite functions, i.e., the production of milk and of beef. Now I think it will be conceded by every stock breeder who has followed these attempts that they have been more or less a failure, because the two purposes which it was intended to combine in the one animal are so distinctly and fundamentally different. To obtain any particular quality, such as milk production, in an animal the breeder must aim at developing and encouraging specific lines of animal individuality, and the attempt to combine and merge together two opposing types of characteristics, such as the ability to give milk and the propensity to pile or flesh has naturally ended in failure. You cannot mix oil and water.

In India, however, we are in a peculiarly fortunate position in regard to cattle breeding in that we are not called upon to combine in one animal diametrically opposite characteristics. On the contrary, we find that the two great requirements of this country from the cattle-breeding point of view, *viz.*, milk and draught, run on parallel lines; so much so that I believe in developing the one along right lines we cannot help advancing the other.

India is overwhelmingly a non-meat-eating country so far as the flesh of the ox is concerned. Consequently beef is not wanted and its production for human food may be left out of count; but India is very much a consumer of milk and milk products, may more, it is largely vegetarian and its people depend for their sustenance upon milk and milk products, and on cereals and pulses grown on cultivated lands, so that what we must produce in this country is an animal the female of which will produce an abundant supply of rich milk, whilst the male can efficiently assist its owner in the cultivation of the soil.

Now let us consider what are the main characteristics of a first class milch cow and see if they are in any way opposed to what we must look for in an efficient plough bullock. The cow must be gentle, maternal, fairly fine boned, not too long in the leg and of massive frame with well-knit symmetrical figure. She must possess great digestive and assimilative ability and have special room for large healthy internal organs; in other words, you want size without height, weight without excessive flesh, frame rather than beef, breeding (which means spirit) rather than bulk, placidity of temper rather than showiness, and the wedge shape in preference to the elephantine type. Surely all these are characteristics of a first class plough or draught bullock as well as of a first class milch cow, and if we admit that the qualities necessary in the one are embodied in the ideal individuality of the other, it behoves the Indian breeder and those who counsel him, to call a halt and to see whether the present policy of breeding for draught only will bear the light of day from an economical standpoint.

Suppose it is granted that a first class field bullock can and does exist, whose female relations give little or no milk, the loss to the country in persisting to breed and rear such a type can only be classed as stupendous, if an equally efficient animal but with milking qualities can be evolved. It may be taken for granted that for every male born a female will also be dropped and the only possible use that female will be to her owner is to produce another uneconomical calf; whereas if in breeding we aim at the dual purpose animal not only can we be certain that the male calf will make a good worker, but his sister will in addition to providing the bullocks for future use give her owner milk worth much gold. We hear a great deal about the reluctance of the cultivator to breed and rear his own bullocks, but the reason is obvious–it does not pay him to do so, and he consequently depends upon the wandering jungle tribes to provide him with cattle. This is bad from many points of view, as the jungle breeder works on haphazard lines, and the rapidly changing agricultural conditions in India will very soon render it impossible for him to produce a first class animal for any purpose; besides until the rearing of cattle is taken up by the *bona fide* cultivator there is little chance of any real improvement being made.

The jungle cattle drover is uneducated and likely to remain so; in short, he cannot be organized or got at to impart him that knowledge necessary to induce him to alter his methods and keep pace with the march of progress. The *Zamindar* and the cultivator on the other hand can be organized, and in a variety of ways they can be influenced. On him then we must depend if we are to regenerate cattle breeding in this country, and this can only be done by demonstrating to cultivators the lines on which cattle breeding can be made to pay. I most strongly contend that outside of breeding on dual purpose lines we cannot do this, but if it can be proved, as I hold it can, to the land owner and the cultivator that by rearing an animal it will give him first class bullocks and heavy milkers, then and then only can he afford to grow fodder crops for cattle breeding and make money at it. From my experience I would say that the average yield of milk of Indian cows all over the country probably does not equal 1,000 lbs. per period of lactation (a fair class of English cow would give 6,000 lbs. per lactation period) and without spending one farthing more on feed than is now expended, but solely by improving the individuality of the animal, this could in a reasonable time be doubled and at the same time the quality of the plough bullocks improved. Consider what it means to the country. Assuming that there are thirty million adult cows in India and taking the value of the increased yield at, say, one anna per lb. means an increase, of £120,000,000 (or say 180 crores of rupees) to the economic wealth of the country in one year. I do not pretend that the above figures of the number of cows in the country is correct–I merely quote it to give an indication of the magnitude of the problem and to show how much it affects the country. It is not necessary to have any expensive schemes for importing European stock in order to develop on dual purpose lines; all that is required is that the breeder should select bulls from the best milkers and keep on doing so. I was shown a herd of Indian cows lately, none of, which were so much used for milk production but all of which were reputed to be the dams of first class working bullocks. On investigation I found that the best milkers had in almost every case produced the best bullocks and this has been my experience generally right through the country. The principle may be applied to either cows or buffaloes where the latter are used for field work, but it is my opinion that on no other lines can cattle breeding in India be put on a sound basis and any permanent improvement be made, because only in this way can the economic laws which govern all such operations be fulfilled. Cattle breeding apart from milk production will not pay the, cultivator, and until the cultivator takes up both cattle breeding and milk production it is almost a hopeless problem to attempt to improve the cattle of India.

The one thing essential before any real progress can be made in improving the cattle of India is that cattle breeding and rearing must be made a paying part of ordinary farming operations. Outside of the dual purpose policy, I do not think this can be done.

Chapter 10

Bulls

The Necessity for a Bull

When there are a number of cows in the dairy, it will be necessary also to keep a good bull to breed from. If there are only one or two cows, and there is a good bull of the same breed in the neighbourhood, the cows can be sent out when they come into season. The charge will not be more than from two to five rupees. In some parts of India there are Government bulls at different stations kept for the benefit of the public, and anyone can have their services for the asking. But if there is no good bull in the neighbourhood, one must be got without delay; for it will never do to have good cows served by inferior bulls.

Every dairy farm should have one or two first class bulls. Unless the cows are put to the bull at the proper time, they will be spoiled for all future dairy use, and when sold will bring in little money. If a cow is not put to the bull when she first comes into season, after her calf is three months old, she is liable to become barren.

It is a great loss to have a cow served by an inferior bull. If a cow is served by a good bull, her milk will increase, but it will be sure to decrease if served by an inferior one. Some good cows are thus spoiled. Then, again, the calf from an inferior bull will be inferior, and will sell for little or nothing.

Whatever breed is selected, great care must be taken that he is of the best type of that breed. It is always best that the bull should be of the same breed as the cows he is to serve if the cows are pure bred. The thorough-bred Montgomery, Sind, Hansi, or Nellore bulls are the best to breed from.

Indian Bulls *versus* English Bulls

It is not advisable to cross Indian cows by English bulls; the progeny rapidly deteriorates. A cross between the best Indian bull and a Shorthorn or Ayrshire cow will prove more satisfactory. If English blood is desired, then cross a good Shorthorn, Ayrshire, or Jersey cow with a first class bull of the best milking strain of one of the following breeds–Montgomery, Sind, Hissar, or Nellore, preferably the Montgomery and Hissar. Select a good bull-calf from this cross, and when he is three years old, use him for covering the cows of the breed his father was. The cross-bred heifers should be mated to a pure bred bull of her father's breed. This method will produce large, strong calves that will prove good milkers, and also retain the good form and characteristics of the Indian breed, and not be as susceptible to disease as the pure English and the first crosses are.

Points in a Good Indian Bull

The height of the bull will depend on his breed. But the larger he is the better. He must be deep and wide in the chest, long and broad in the back, and round in the barrel, well ribbed up and strong in the shoulders and limbs, and have massive but not very long legs; large joints, and legs fairly apart to support the body; compact and solid-looking carcass; short face, with large, prominent eyes, set far apart, and broad forehead and muzzle. His neck must be short and stout, rising well over the withers into a large hump. The head should be carried erect. The dewlap should be long, but the ears should not be very long. The sheath should not be very long and pendulous.

Age

It is a very serious mistake to use an immature bull for breeding purposes. The progeny of such a bull will be weak and very hard to rear, and very often the mother's milk will decrease very perceptibly. A bull should never be used before he is three years old, nor after he is eight years old. Some bulls are productive until they are ten years old. Some bulls are used when they are only two years of age but this is a very bad practice. Very often very young and also inferior bulls prove unproductive.

Care and Attention

A bull needs proper care and attention. Some people let him

loose to wander about at pleasure, and pick up what he can in the way of food, and never think of giving him any shelter or special attention. If the bull is not looked after, he will be ruined. He must be sheltered at nights and from the midday sun and heavy rains, and must have good wholesome food regularly.

Food

He should be fed twice a day, once at 6 A.M., and again at sunset. The following is sufficient for two meals for a large Montgomery or Sind bull, but an Ongole or Hissar bull will need probably 2 lb. more of gram and less of bran, grass and chaff.

Gram (broken)	2 lb.
Mustard oilcake (khullie)	1 lb.
Wheat-bran (*bhoosi*)	3 lb.
Green grass	8 to 10 lb.
Chaff (*bhoosa*) or straw	16 to 20 lb.
Salt	2 ounces
Sulphur	½ ounce

Besides this quantity of food, wherever it is possible, the bull should be tied out to graze. When there is no grass lands for the bull to graze on, he should be allowed as much extra grass or straw as he will eat. Young *jowar* and Indian-corn stalks and leaves should be given instead of straw when procurable.

When green food is not available additional *bhoosa*, straw and 2 lb. of wheat-bran or 1 lb. of gram must be allowed.

Utensils, House and Grooming

The feeding utensils and the house should be kept scrupulously clean, and the animal regularly groomed and washed, and allowed plenty of exercise. It is not at all a bad plan to give him some light work every day, such as drawing water or working the cart to remove the refuse, but he must not be in the least tired out. This will keep him fit and docile.

Fat

A bull should never be allowed to become very fat, but should always be in good tough condition.

Keeping Him Separate

Some people allow the bull to run with the cows in the herd. If the bull be a large one and very quiet, this may be done without harm, but most bulls are best kept apart, and should be allowed the company of the cow only when she needs his services.

Serving

When a cow is in heat she should be tied up and the bull put to her. Two servings are enough. This will conserve the bull's strength, which is wasted when he is allowed to run after the cow, or the cow is allowed to jump about.

Over-Serving

Bulls are generally spoiled by over-serving. A bull should not be allowed to serve more than one cow a week. An occasional deviation from this rule will not hurt him if he is allowed to serve each cow only once or twice. If a bull be used too much, he will become barren, or else the calves from him will be weak and die early. This is one of the chief defects in *bazaar bulls* and many of the bulls kept for serving the cows of the public.

The Sire

(*The Journal of Dairying*)

A good male should head the herd. If heifer calves worth while are to be raised to replenish the herd, a poor bull is more expensive in the long run than a few poor cows, and should not be taken as a gift. No one can afford to use a "scrub" and no progressive dairyman will use one. The kind of bull used advertises the energy and intelligence of his owner. It is wise to avoid buying even heifers from the man who uses a "scrub" bull, or a bull of beef breeding.

The problem of selecting a good sire is not always an easy one. At the present time the majority of breeders do not keep accurate records of the production of their cows, and hence are not able to give accurate information to purchasers of their bull-calves. It sometimes happens that bulls from high-producing dams fail to transmit this quality to their offspring, but they are much more likely to do so than bulls from low-producing dams. In using young bulls this risk must always be taken. For this reason it is especially important that one should look carefully into the records of the dam and the sire's dam before purchasing. When possible, it is desirable to purchase a seven or eight years old bull which has proved his merit by the high production of his daughters, provided he is in good health. The majority of men object to handling aged bulls because often they are vicious. For this reason few bulls are kept until their heifers are in milk and their productive capacity determined. Until this time the sire's real value is unknown. Many a good bull which would have made his owner famous has been slaughtered at an early age.

The selection of the herd bull is of the greatest importance, because he is at least half the herd from the breeding standpoint. His influence on the characteristics of every calf born in the herd is as great as that of the dam of the calf; and if he is a pure-bred animal used on grade cows, his influence will be more than half because his transmitting powers in breed characteristics will be stronger.

Chapter 11

Bullocks

Bullocks and Buffaloes are the only animals used in the plough in India. They are also very largely used in the cart and carriage. Very often, keeping one's own bullocks and cart is a great saving and convenience.

The points in a good bullock are the same as those in a good bull–only, bullocks are not so heavy as bulls, and are much more active and fiery, and walk faster. When their tails or hips are touched, they run.

The creamy white are considered to be generally not very strong, but some creamy white bulls are found to be perfect in every respect. Very large dewlaps and very much loose skin under the stomach of bullocks and very large pendulous ears are considered signs of weakness.

When a bull-calf is castrated, his form undergoes somewhat of a change, and he sometimes looks like a cow. A calf should be castrated when he is between 6 and 10 months old.

Food

Working bullocks should have the same quality of food as bulls, and the quantities fixed according to their size and amount of work they are required to perform. Instead of two meals, three should be given: one at daybreak, the second at 1 P.M., and the last at sunset when they are tied up for the night. They should never be fed immediately before or after hard work. An interval of two hours should be allowed between the meals and work. When a bullock is not regular and hard work his food should be proportionateiy reduced. A bullock should be kept in good tough condition but never allowed to get fat.

Grooming and Cleaning

Bullocks need to be properly groomed every day and kept perfectly clean, and their utensils and house should be kept as clean as those of cows. Bullocks should not be exposed to the midday sun and heavy rains and cold sharp winds. When obliged to keep them outside in the cold they should have *jhools* put on them.

Water

Bullocks and bulls should have plenty of clean drinking-water.

Rearing Bullocks

When a calf is reared for the plough, and especially the cart, he should be allowed the greater portion of his mother's milk, for the first three months at least, and, in addition, a liberal supply of good wholesome prepared food. After he is three months of age he should be given a good quantity of ground oats, gram, oilcake, wheat-bran and green food. The beautiful animals we sometimes see in carriages up-country were never deprived of any portion of their mothers' milk, and were well cared for and fed from the beginning. They should be kept loose in fields or paddocks and not kept tied.

Chapter 12

Dry Cows

Selling Dry Cows

Some persons think dry cows a great trouble and expense to keep, and as soon as their cows stop milking they sell them. Unless a cow is an inferior one, or has been spoiled, has blind teats, is diseased, or has become barren, she should not be sold because she has run dry. As has been said, a good cow will amply repay her owner if kept till she calves again.

Keeping Dry Cows that are in calf is not a great expense. Dry ones sell for a quarter the price of cows in full milk. If it is certain she is in calf and has been served by a good bull she will fetch half the price of cows in milk. The cost of keeping a dry cow until she calves will not exceed the difference in price between a dry one and one in full milk, and the owner will be fully repaid by the improved quality and quantity of the milk, due to proper care and management. A cow should milk up to three months of the time of calving again.

A good cow giving from 20 to 24 lb. of milk will cost, in Kolkata, about Rs. 300 or Rs. 350. She will milk for 300 days, and average 12 lb. of milk a day. The yield for 300 days will be 3,600 lb. The value of this at 6 1b. per rupee is Rs. 600. The cost of food and keep for the period will be Rs. 300. Now if the cow is properly managed, she will yield the following profit, if sold when dry–

Dr.	
Purchase of cow	Rs. 350
Cost of food, etc.	Rs. 300
	Total Rs. 650

Cr.	
Value of milk	Rs. 600
Value of calf at ten months	Rs. 60
Sale of cow to butcher	Rs. 70
	Total Rs. 730
	Expenditure Rs. 650
	Profit Rs. 80

If kept till next calving-

Dr.	
Purchase of cow	Rs. 350
Cost of food. etc., for ten months	Rs. 300
Extra cost for four months when dry	Rs. 40
	Total Rs. 690

Cr.	
Value of milk	Rs. 600
Value of calf	Rs. 60
Value of cow when she calves again	Rs. 350
	Total Rs. 1,010
	Expenditure Rs. 690
	Profit Rs. 320

So we see that to keep a cow for the second year will yield more than three times the profit that she yields if kept only one year. Of course, this presupposes proper management. It will never pay a dairyman in India to fatten cows for the butcher. Every cow he has to sell is so much loss, and every cow he is able to keep and breed from is so much gain. The chief reason why so many dairymen in cities and towns fail in their business is that they allow their calves to die, and spoil their cows and sell them to butchers. This is invariably the result of bad management and leaving things in the hands of the servants.

Advantage

"It is advantageous to buy a cow before she calves, as you then get the whole of her milk; you have also the management of her before and after calving, and if she be in skilful hands, she will give more milk than she would do if mismanaged."

"It is also well to get her accustomed to her attendants and her stall before she calves, as any change of quarters afterwards will male her feet, and this will at once tell on her milk. If the calf is not very young, any check of this kind will lessen her milk permanently. So it often happens that the purchaser of a cow in milk complains that the cow does not give as much milk as he was led to suppose she did, the reason being that the milk has been lessened by the fretting of the cow on changing hands. The rest and care will make the cow a better milker when she calves."–*Cows in India.*

Food

Some cows continue to give full milk until they are four or five months in calf again, some lessen their milk soon after becoming pregnant. Between the sixth and seventh month from the birth of her calf a cow will begin to give less milk; as the milk lessens the food should be gradually reduced. "It is difficult to decide when to begin to reduce a cow's food from full feed to the spare diet of a dry cow. When a cow is in calf, and is going off her milk, and you have no other cow giving milk or need her milk for butter, continue to feed her up; but if you have sufficient milk from other cows, or if the quantity she gives is not worth the cost other food, it is better to put her on spare diet and leave her calf loose to drink what she gives. It will strengthen the calf and do the cow good."–*Cows in India.*

The reduction of food should be gradual. First stop the oilcake; after some days stop the *kallaie;* after another few days reduce the gram and bran. But give larger quantities of green grass and *bhoosa.* Dry cows must not have oilcake, cotton-seed, or any kind of food that fattens much. Fat in a cow is serious defect; it makes her liable to slipping her calf, and also becoming barren.

A dry cow should have plenty of grazing during the day, and some cut green grass, hay, or *bhoosa*, with 2 lb. of wheat-bran and 1 lb. of ground gram and 1 ounce of salt, to munch during the night; but on no account give her any mustard oilcake or other heating food. If ground gram is not given, give 4 lb. wheat-bran instead of 2 lb. She should be kept in fair condition to within a few weeks of her time of calving, when she will pick up of herself, if she gets a sufficient quantity of green grass. If green grass is not obtainable she should be allowed 2 lb. bran and ½ lb. gram twice a day, mixed with cut straw or *bhoosa* and sufficient water. If, on the other hand, the cow is starved, and allowed to get into bad condition the calf will be weak and sickly.

Over-Feeding

"Over-feeding when a cow is not in milk makes the food run to fat, and if a cow's food once begins to do this, it will continue to do so when she is fed up after calving, and in a short time she will be fit only for the butcher,–though she may have a fat udder and a large belly, her milk will be scanty. But if the extra food comes at calving with the fresh milk, all the food goes to milk, as the system has become accustomed to spare diet, and being healthy her muscles will improve, but she will not put on fat. If she is allowed to get fat before calving, her calf will he born puny."–*Cows in India.*

The reason why so many calves are still-born, or die soon afterbirth, is that the cows are allowed to become too fat. Over-feeding and want of exercise will cause a cow to grow fat. Heating food, such as oilcake and certain grains, will cause the cow to throw off and wish to go to the bull again. Sometimes a cow will, without throwing off, get into heat and take the bull; this will injure the calf and cause miscarriage.

The calf of a fat, over-fed cow will be small and weak or deformed, and not live long.

Young bulls and barren cows, and also cows that are in heat, will worry cows that are in calf and injure them.

Exercise

Cows that are in calf must not be kept tied up all the day. They should be allowed to graze in the compound or fields near the house, or else they should be tied out in some open place with ropes at least

40 feet long. Exercise is absolutely necessary for cows that are in calf. If they do not get it, they will suffer at the time of calving.

Care

Cows in calf should have plenty of exercise, but great care should be taken that they do not fight with other cows or meet with any accident. They must not be allowed to jump or run, and they must not be driven fast or jerked. They should be groomed and washed gently and kept clean and dry; cows during pregnancy are very delicate, and if neglected or hurt will become ill or slip the calf. Purgatives and strong medicines are contra-indicated.

Protection from Disease

Every care must be taken to keep pregnant cows away from cows that have had abortion and from all sick animals.

Cleanliness about their food, water, utensils, and house is just as essential as when they are milking.

Time of Pregnancy

The time a cow is in calf is about 290 days; age and condition of health make a slight difference. The calf quickens between the fourth and fifth month.

Selling Dry Cows to Butchers

It is a great loss to the country and a crime to allow good cows to go to the butcher. Large numbers of really good milch cows are brought to the cities and towns by cattle dealers and sold to milkmen. These milkmen, who are mostly illiterates, allow the calves to die or else sell them soon to butchers, and force the cows to give as much milk as they can. This forcing is done by special feeding and by the cruel process of *phooka*. The cows give milk for five to eight months and become fat. They are not allowed to get into calf, but are sold to the butcher as soon as they stop giving sufficient milk to pay the cost of their keep. In this way thousands of valuable cows and calves are sacrificed every year by the city milkmen.

Formerly the milkmen used to sell these cows directly to butchers, but now they sell them to the cattle dealers from whom the butchers buy them. The dealer sells a cow in milk to a milkman and takes the dry cow in part payment, and then sells her to the butcher.

The dealer, as a rule, takes the dry cow for Rs. 30 or Rs. 40, and sells her for Rs. 40 or Rs. 60 to the butcher. These milk men will tell people that they do not sell their calves or cows to butchers, but send them back to their country to breed from; this is all a trick–the dealers never send the cows to their country. They are sold to butchers or sent to Rangoon and Singapore for slaughter.

The Government and Municipalities should step in to prevent good cows being slaughtered. No cow or heifer of milking breeds should be allowed to be slaughtered, until it is proved that she is barren. This can be proved only if she has not got into calf within two years from the time she had her last calf.

How to Dispose of Dry Cows and Young Calves

When people have cows of good breeds that have stopped giving milk and calves for sale, if they would advertise in the daily newspapers they would find many persons ready to buy them for breeding. There are Europeans and Indians living in the mofussil who have facilities for keeping a few good cows, and if they could get cows of good breeds that have stopped milking for Rs. 50 and Rs. 60 each, they would be glad to buy them. If a cow is bought for Rs. 60, and kept for, say, ten months before she calves, the cost of her food and keep for this period would not exceed Rs. 80. When she calves, her price will be from Rs. 200 to Rs. 300.

Dairymen and other people who keep cows should be willing to sell their dry cows to such people rather than to butchers, and they should be willing to take the same prices from these people that dealers and butchers would give them.

If a cow is in calf people would be willing to pay more money for them, for there is always a certain risk in buying dry cows not in calf, as they may not get into calf for a long while. If people who have dry cows for sale would be reasonable and ask the price butchers offer, they would find no difficulty whatever in finding good homes for their cows. Good calves could be disposed of in the same way.

Sellers should be honest and state how long the cow has been milking, how long the calf has been dead, if the teats are all right, if the cow has been ruined by the *gowallas*, if she has any sickness, and if she gives any trouble in milking; for a cow that bas been spoiled or is unhealthy is not fit for breeding.

Chapter 13

Management of Cows When Calving

Little needs to be done for a cow before the time of calving, beyond attending to her food, rest, and exercise.

Signs of the Time

When a cow is within a few days of calving, her shape will undergo a change: she wil become hollow just beneath the hip bones, and her stomach will appear as if sunk down towards the chest; in the case of an old cow it is very evident that a great change has taken place in the position of the calf. Some animals evince uneasiness and irritation of the bowels and bladder by the constant motion of the tail, and by the ineffectual attempts made to dung; the vagina becomes loosened and increased in size, and a white or pale straw-coloured glairy discharge exudes from it some two or three weeks before the time. As soon as this change is observed, the cow must not be sent out to graze, but must be kept at home in order that the event may not be unduly hurried from any unforeseen cause. If a cow calves away from home, she runs the risk of catching a chill. Some cows calve very quickly, even the very day the change is observed, while others may not do so for a week or more. Keeping them quiet has very beneficial effect upon them. About ten or fifteen days before calving, the udder increases, and sometimes becomes full of milk, and the milk-vein is distended. A cow in this state is very liable to take a chill; she should be kept dry and away from draughts, and should not be bathed, specially during winter.

If the udder is very much enlarged and the milk-vein distended, it should be fomented with warm water in which some Epsom salt or boracic or Jaye's fluid has been dissolved and it should be emptied every morning and evening. Unless this is done, inflammation of the udder may set in, and both cow and calf suffer much. If the cow is once milked, she must be milked regularly every day, and every drop extracted. After milking, rub some camphorated mustard oil on the udder. The cow's vagina should be washed with slightly warm water in which a little phenyle or Jaye's fluid has been dissolved. After washing, wipe thoroughly. The room or stall must be thoroughly washed with a strong solution of phenyle and water and dried and sufficient quantity of bedding provided.

Labour Approaching

"An hour or two before the event, the face of the cow will bear an anxious look; the eyes will be bright and staring and hollow, indicative of pain. As soon as the cow shows these signs, she should be taken into her house and kept quiet; some straw should be spread on the floor, and she should be given a good supply of soft green grass to amuse herself and keep her from fretting. The straw must be thoroughly clean and disinfected. Her keeper should remain close at hand, but be careful not to disturb her unnecessarily, nor sit and watch her from where she can see him. She will eat a little at times when out of pain. When she begins to sit down and get up, as if uneasy, the man should stay with her until the calf is born, and afterwards he should prevent her from getting up until the calf is quite clear of its mother."–*Cows in India.*

Progress of Labour

The actual progress of labour becomes evident by the protrusion of the membranes, or "bag of water " as it is termed, which breaks the animal lies down, and, after a while, turns flat on her side, generally the left. The fore feet of the calf may now be seen protruding through the vulva; and, as labour advances, the head comes forth closely applied over the fore feet, with the chin resting on the knees, and the back of the calf parallel to that of the cow. After the head makes its appearance there is a short respite of some two or three minutes, and the trunk and hind extremities, stretched at full length, are pushed out by the expulsive efforts of the uterus assisted by the diaphragm and abdominal muscles. A few seconds after the birth of the calf the cow sits up, and then, rising on her legs, commences to lick her calf, which she does incessantly for some time, the calf while lying still, stretched out and gasping. Gradually it raises its head, draws its fore feet under it, and begins to make ineffectual efforts to get on its legs, which it eventually succeeds in doing. It then totters about, by degrees attains firmness on its legs, and after a short time is able to support its body steadily."–*A Manual of Indian Cattle and Sheep*.

Assistance Needed

In most cases no assistance whatever is needed. Nature accomplishing her course with perfect safety to mother and young. Occasionally a cross-birth may occur, and surgical assistance be necessary. In such cases a doctor should be called in at once and the calf should not be pulled to make the position still more difficult. This is usual with the servants and should be guarded against carefully.

At the moment of calving most of the people know what to do, and are good nurses if the birth be a natural one. Where they fail is in the management before and after birth.

Treatment of the Cow After the Birth of the Calf

When the cow and calf have been attended to the people ordinarily give half a pound of *gurh* (molasses), half a pound of dried ginger, and two ounces of *huldi* (turmeric). The ginger and *huldi* are well ground, and mixed with the *gurh* and some wheat-bran, and the cow is given half the mixture at once, as it helps to clear away the after-birth, and reduce the after-pains which trouble and weaken some well-bred cows very much; many of the best milkers are very delicate, and suffer much at the time of calving. The remainder of the mixture of ginger and *gurh* are given about six hours afterwards.

Great care is needed to prevent the cow's vagina and the calf's navel from becoming sore and getting blown by flies. They must be washed every day with phenyle and warm water, and, after drying them thoroughly with a clean soft cloth, the following ointment must be applied: Sweet oil or pure vaseline, four ounces; camphor, one ounce; spirits of turpentine, two ounces. This must be done every morning and evening for a week or ten days.

Immediately after the calf is born, its mouth, throat and nostrils should be cleaned, its navel painted with tincture of iodine after washing with phenyle and water, and a ligature put two inches from the skin to prevent infection. The mother must not be allowed to lick the navel. After this camphorated vaseline may be applied.

Drink and Food

"Care must be taken that the cow has nothing to drink, and that she has a warm coat thrown over her, or she is very apt to catch cold particularly during winter for the first hours succeeding the birth of the calf. If she is doing well, the less she is disturbed the better; but if her eyes become glassy and of a steel colour when the light is thrown on them, and the hollows above them deepen, she is in pain, and about four hours after the birth she should have a hot bran-mash, rather sloppy, which will fill and warm her inside, and quell the pain. This should be continued for the first three days, as it assists the milk to come, keeps her inside warm, and opens her bowels. For the first week she should have warm water to drink; this is a point to be very careful about, as a draught of cold water will chill her, and may produce respiratory complaints, swollen udder and inflamed nipples–most troublesome complaints, resulting in the cow drying up–and she suffers so much pain that she will not allow herself to be milked, nor her calf to suck."–*Cows in India*. (See Part 2, Chapter 3).

For the first week the cow must not have any other food than plenty of soft green grass and two to four pounds of wheat-bran with one ounce of salt, and one ounce of pounded *huldi* (turmeric) added to it. This must be given twice or three times a day. For the first three days no straw should be given, and for the first week no rich food, as it may cause inflammation of the udder.

It must be remembered that cows that are large milkers are unnatural cows; they are like cultivated plants, very delicate. A common cow that gives only enough milk for her calf may stand neglect, but a good milker will go wrong in no time.

Illness

Anything wrong with a cow at such a time must be promptly attended to. (*See* Part 2, Chapter 3).

Falling of the Womb

See Part 2, Chapter 3.

Milking

About an hour or so after a cow has calved and the after-birth is expelled she should be milked, and the calf set to suck. The calf should be kept with the mother, and allowed to suck her frequently; the sucking will open the milk-vessels, and bring the milking machinery into play; the calf being hungry will suck hard, and draw off pain from the cow. But the cow must be milked regularly three times a day after calving, and every drop of milk extracted each time. An hour before she is milked the calf should be separated from the mother. On the third day the real flow of milk sets in, the udder increases, and the milk is quite fit to use for puddings and butter; the butter will be large in quantity, and rich in colour and flavour. The milk should not be given to babies until the calf is three weeks old. After the seventh day, and until the end of the first month after calving, the milk will not produce much butter. When the calf is allowed to be with the mother, great care is needed lest the cow crush the calf. The best method is to allow the calf to suck for half an hour or an hour, and then shut it up in its own room for three hours, when the calf is let loose to suck again for another half an hour or so, and again put it away. This may be continued throughout the day and night for the first three weeks or month.

Chapter 14

Calves: Their Value, Management and House

Value of Calves

The value of a calf depends much upon its breed and the condition it is in, just as a thorough-bred colt is of greater value than a common one. The price of a year-old calf of the common village cattle will be anything from Rs. 8 to Rs. 12; and a two-year old one from Rs. 12 to Rs. 15. The better class village calves will sell from Rs. 20 to Rs. 30 when a year old, and double that when two years old. Calves of pure-bred Montomery, Sind, Hissar, and Ongole cattle will fetch as much as from Rs. 50 to Rs. 70 when ten months or a year old, and Rs. 100 to Rs. 200 when two years old. The price of a female calf is always less than the price of a bull-calf or bullock-calf.

The price of a cow is highest after she has had her first; calf, and the price of a bull as well as a bullock is highest when he is between three and five years of age.

Some calves are inferior and not worth the trouble and expense of rearing; such should be sold for what they will fetch as soon as their mothers stop milking and refuse to allow them to suck. But if a calf is a good one, it should be kept to replenish the stock. The cost of its keep and food will not exceed its value.

Food and Care

It is no economy to starve or neglect the calf. If it gets out of condition and becomes sickly, its growth and development will be affected, and its value materially lessened. Whereas if it dies, the mother's supply of milk is sure to decrease and the cow liable to go dry. A calf should never be deprived of its mother's milk. For the first month or so after its birth the calf will not eat anything, and if not allowed sufficient of its another's milk its development will be seriously hampered. The calf should be allowed to suck its mother every three hours between five in the morning and nine at night. The cow should be milked at 5 A.M., 12 midday, and at 6 P.M. for the first month, and the milk drawn and then the calf allowed to suck. At the other hours she should not be milked but the calf allowed to drink all it can. After the first month the cow should be milked in the morning and after that the calf allowed to be with her for a couple of hours; the cow should be again milked at midday and the calf allowed to remain with the mother for an hour. At five or six in the evening the cow should be milked again and then the calf allowed to suck for two hours. This should be done until the calf is three months old and can eat properly, then it need remain with the mother for an hour in the morning and an hour in the evening only after she is milked.

The English method of hand feeding the calves is not ordinarily adopted by Indians, moreover the Indian cow will not allow her calf to be taken from her. If it is done, she will never milk as well or for as long a period as she would if she were allowed her calf. English cows have generations of training at the back of them, and the separation from their calves does not injure them. It will take generations of training to make the Indian cow do without her calf. It is not advisable for anyone to try it. If properly treated, the cow will give more milk with her calf than she will do without it. And the calf will not take more from the mother than would be given to it if fed from the pail.

The calf must be given some extra food besides what it gets from its mother. When the calf is three weeks old some gram, wheat or oats should be finely ground and soaked, and then slightly boiled and given to it three times a day. And to this one ounce of finely ground linseed meal. Some finely cut soft *doob* grass should be given. But on no account give the little thing dry bran and straw, as so many people do. Until the calf is three months old special care must be taken about its food, shelter and cleanliness. Neglect at this time means disaster. For the first three weeks or a month it will not eat much, but if given food regularly it will only nibble at it and soon learn to eat and like it. It must be taught to eat by putting the food into its mouth and holding its mouth up.

As it grows bigger, increase the quantity of ground gram and give some sweet linseed oilcake and wheat-bran. Mustard-seed oilcake is positively injurious to young calves under four months of age. A little salt and sulphur and *gurh-jaggery* should be given to the calf from the beginning. Over-feeding is bad; half a pound of ground gram and two ounces of linseed meal, or half a pound of ground oats or wheat with linseed meal, is enough to begin with. Then add half a pound of good wheat-bran, and in place of linseed meal give quarter of a pound of good sweet linseed oilcake. These, quantities should be given to the calf three times a day until it is two months old. From two to three months of age gradually increase the food. A liberal supply of tender green grass should be always allowed. Pure drinking-water should be given at *libitum*. When a calf is between three and four months old, it is advisable to give it half a pound of ground gram, one pound of wheat-bran, and half pound of linseed oilcake or quarter pound of mustard oilcake in each meal three times a day.

At six months of age a Montgomery, or Sind calf should get half pound of mustard oilcake, three pounds of wheat-bran, and one pound of ground gram or crushed oats in the morning, and the same quantity in the evening. At midday it should be allowed out to graze or given plenty of grass, hay, or silage.

The best time to feed the calves is after the cows have been milked and the calves separated from them. Regularity in feeding is indispensable.

Tying up Calves

Little calves should never be tied up; if tied they should not be kept long. They must be kept loose in a shed or room with an enclosure or paddock where they may run about.

House

The calves must be kept separate from the other cattle, and their room kept clean, dry, and warm, and properly ventilated. The flooring of the calves' room must be *pucca*, and thoroughly scrubbed every morning and evening. A calf needs at least 5 feet by 6 feet of room. Dry and clean straw should be spread on the floor for them.

On no account should calves be allowed to sit on wet or damp ground or grass. In the cold weather nights they should be kept in a warm room or pen.

Shelter from Sun and Rain

Calves should not be much exposed to the midday sun, or rain, and should be sheltered from the cold (north and east) winds. They are very delicate creatures, and any neglect may prove fatal.

Ticks and Lice

Calves must be kept absolutely free from ticks and lice. Regular brushing will keep them free from vermin. Little calves should sparingly be bathed and dried up completely. 1f troubled with lice and ticks, apply some of the liniment for destroying vermin (*see* Recipes).

Older Calves

When bull-calves are six months old they should be tied up and fed. Heifers should be tied up and fed when they are four or five months old, but not kept tied all the day. Male calves should be very liberally fed; the quantity of their food should be gradually and continually increased, until at eighteen months of age they receive the same quantity and quality of food as prescribed for bulls.

Heifers need special attention; very often they are neglected and receive neither proper food nor shelter, consequently they are small and deformed, and are unfit for milking or breeding purposes. Then again, some heifers are so highly fed that they become barren. In many cases all the efforts of the owners have failed to make the animals productive. These heifers come into season and take the bull, but never get into calf. They have been spoiled by overheating and too much food. Heifers should be kept in good condition, but never allowed to grow very fat. They should be fed on the same kind of food as milch cows, but should not be allowed so much oilcake or grain and on no account any cotton-seed. Good green grass, wheat-bran, *bhoosa* and chopped straw should be given in abundance. The food should be prepared in the same way as food for milch cows. Some salt and an unlimited supply of pure drinking-water are essential to the animal's health.

Careful Treatment

A great deal of care is needed in the management of calves. The temper and habits of cows and bullocks depend a great deal upon the treatment they have received when calves. If one wants good milch cows, then he ought to observe the following what the *American Farmer* says:

Treat the Cows Kindly

"Here is a bit of gospel truth which should be heeded, especially by dairymen. Animals, like human beings, will respond to kindness, and on a dairy farm this is one of the greatest essentials to success. You cannot begin too early in training your calves to come at your call, and to submit to handling and petting. Accustom them to familiarity with persons, but never permit them to be vexed or irritated, if you do not want them to become ill-natured cows. While good blood is of the greatest importance, still if not properly trained the highest satisfaction will not be attained. A good animal may be spoiled by bad management. Good feed, good care, and petting will naturally aid in securing good results."

This is very true about heifers. There are cows that would not allow themselves to be tied or touched, and are as wild as jungly cattle. Though of good breeds they are unfit for domestic use. Their bad habits are attributable to nothing else but bad management when calves.

Male calves that are intended for the plough or cart should not be treated like the heifers. The less they are tied up and petted and handled the better; their backs or tails should not be touched. Handling and petting bull-calves makes them very tame and slow in harness, and considerably lessens their value.

Why So Many Calves Die

A large number of calves die from sheer neglect and mismanagement. They are deprived of their mothers' milk, and insufficient and unwholesome food is given to them; they are exposed to sudden changes of weather, and not sheltered from the cold and damp at night, or heat in the day; they are allowed to become covered with lice and ticks, and their houses are kept unclean. Milkmen in cities and towns, and servants of private owners, are the principal offenders in this matter. Unless the calves are given special attention the servant will neglect and kill them.

If the calf is cared for and properly reared, it will help the cow to give more milk and milk for a longer time, and the calf will repay all that is spent on its care and food.

Chapter 15

Points in a Good Calf

"A good bull-calf should have loose skin running from his chin down his dewlap and round his chest and along his belly; his eyes should be far apart, and his forehead broad; has nose short and turned up; his joints large and looking swollen. The size of the joints is an indication of his eventual growth, and the better bred he is the more ungainly will his joints be. The shorter his neck the greater will be his strength. His hair should be soft, long, and rather curly. If he is in good health his nose will be wet and shining. An ill-bred calf will have a narrow head, very long ears, small eyes rather close together, long neck, small joints, and legs tapering away at the feet like a goat's."–*Cows in India.*

"A good cow-calf should have much the same points as a bull-calf, but her head will not be so broad or her neck so short; and instead of the long dewlap, she should have, if of a good milking breed, lots of yellow wrinkled skin between her legs where the udder will be in time to come, and she will have well-developed teats, even when only a few hours old; and the best milkers will always have silky hair."–*Cows in India.*

The breed of the calf will make some difference in its appearance. A Hissar and Nellore calf will be larger and broader and have larger joints than will a Montgomery and Sind calf.

Chapter 16

Castrating Calves

Castrating When Young

In Europe, calves as a rule are castrated between the first and the third month after birth. The advantage of the operation at this early age consists in the improvement of the animal in form; size and the propensity to fatten, while it also renders him docile and generally useful as a working bullock. The people here, on the contrary, wait still longer-of course which is not desirable.

Mode of Castration

Calves formerly used to be castrated without cutting the scrotum at all. The bull used to be thrown down and its four legs tied together: then the scrotum was drawn out and freely handled for a few minutes to relax it; after which a rope or string used to be tied on to the cord above the gland, and then with a stout wooden roller, about 15 inches in length and 1½ inch in diameter, the glands used to be placed over some hard object and hammered and crushed. A man used to sit and press the gland tightly till it burst within its sack or the scrotum, between the fingers of both his hands, and kneaded it well till it became broken up into a soft pulp. The other gland was next drawn and crushed in like manner and a little *huldi* (turmeric) was lastly smeared over the scrotum. This is a cruel method and is not much in vogue now; the method nowadays practised is Castration by Burrdizzo's method which is perhaps the best method at present known. By this the cords are simply crushed without cutting open the skin. No further treatment is ever necessary excepting irrigation of cold water and the application of tincture of iodine to the parts. The animal is well in ten days.

Effect of This Process

There is no wound or subsequent discharge and disturbance with flies, etc., is the case after cutting. The scrotum although swells slightly but in ten days or a fortnight the swelling becomes absorbed and looks as nothing had happened. This process of castrating is never attended with any danger, nor is it so painful as the cutting process. The animals further retain their masculine form to a certain extent. When a young calf is castrated, it soon loses its masculine form, and as it grows larger it looks somewhat like a cow; but when the cords are crushed the change in form is not so great, though the animal may not become as large as it would have if it had been castrated.

Great Care in the Operation

When the cords are crushed, great care must be taken that they are very thoroughly crushed up, otherwise the animal will occasionally prove troublesome among the cows. To avoid this, each cord should be crushed in two places with an inter-space of about an inch between the two. When the calf is castrated by other method care must be taken that the sore is not fly-blown or allowed to fester.

Proper Time to Castrate

A calf should be castrated when it is between six and ten months old.

The Evil of Late Castration

The evil of late castration consists in the young bulls being allowed to roam at large with the cows. People here never think of separating the bulls from the cows. Even if there be a good bull in the herd, he is over-reached by those young bulls, from their lightness of carcass and activity in serving the cows.

Chapter 17

Taking the Bull

A Very Important Matter

This is a critical moment with owners of cows, because it is a matter of very great importance, and any mistake at this time will very seriously affect the profit to be derived from the cow.

Before putting a cow to the bull, the owner must be certain that she is not already in calf. If a cow in calf be put to the bull, it will very seriously injure her and will be certain to cause a miscarriage of the young one, of course generally the bulls never care for pregnant or dry cows which are not in season. Many people think that a cow in calf will not show any signs of being in heat. This is a mistake. It is known that cows that have progressed as far as six or seven months in pregnancy worry other cows by jumping on them. But such a mistake as putting a cow in calf to the bull can be very effectually prevented.

Early Months of Pregnancy

In the early months of pregnancy it is difficult to decide if a cow is or is not in calf. It is most necessary to know for certain, both to her lying fallow when she ought to be in calf, and also to prevent her being put to the bull when she is already in calf and causing much mischief.

Signs of Pregnancy

The most certain sign of a cow carrying is a thick and sticky discharge from the vagina, and which adheres to the tail and is called "Show". In the absence of this, it is probable that she is not in calf. In the later months, a cow's condition is quite evident from the size of her abdomen.

Between the fourth and fifth months of pregnancy, it can be ascertained with some amount of certainty that a cow is in calf. The calf may be felt by putting the palm of the hands hard against the right flank of the cow when a hard lump will bound against the abdomen and be felt by the hands; or when a bucket of cold water is dashed against the right flank or drunk by the cow the calf kicks and a convulsive motion may be observed in the flank by looking at it from behind; if the open hand is then laid upon the space between the flank and the udder this motion may be distinctly felt.

When a Cow Comes into Season

A cow generally comes into season and is put to the bull three months after the birth of her last calf. But after this, it is very injurious to the cow to neglect the wants of Nature. If she calls for the bull and is neglected, she may become barren.

Rich food and over-feeding have the effect of bringing the cow into season before the proper time for it.

Some heifers take the bull when they are eighteen months old. Others again, do not come into season until they are about three years old. A heifer, if properly led and cared for, should take the bull when she is two years and three months old.

Some cows come into season in three months from the time they have last calved. These have a calf every twelve or thirteen months. Others, again, milk for six or eight months before they take the bull; it has been seen that the Hansi milked for twelve months before she took bull.

The Symptoms of Coming into Season

The symptoms of coming into season are, abatement of milk and restlessness. The cow will be frequently dunging, staling, and bellowing, but some cows do not bellow. Her tail will be in constant motion, and she will have no appetite. The vagina will appear red and inflamed, and a transparent discharge will sometimes flow from it. If in the field, the cow will be riding other cows; if tied, she will stamp with her feet and pull at her rope. Some become very savage, and will butt. Others, again, show their state but little, often doing no more than lowing gently or with only slight vaginal discharge; these latter are apt to be neglected, as their state is not soon observed.

The Time a Cow Remains in Season

These symptoms last only for a day or two (more or less) and the cow should be put to the bull immediately, afterwards she should be given a cold bath and kept on low diet for a month or two. Time is an object. If the cow has taken the bull and not become pregnant, the above mentioned symptoms will return in three weeks, and continue to do so until she does conceive. A fat, over-fed cow will want to go out to the bull time after time until she is in calf. Such a cow must be reduced in condition before she will become pregnant.

Troublesome Cows

If a cow remains ten months without getting into calf, she should be sent out altogether to remain with the other cattle in the field, grazing and feeding with them. The company and change of air, food and exercise may have the desired effect. If a cow does not come into season when she should, give her some heating food, *e.g.*, mustard oilcake in bigger quantities or gram.

When a cow comes into season but fails to conceive-even after she has been shown to the bull for several times-she should be examined by a Veterinary Surgeon, preferably as sometimes there is found a layer of gelatinous substance, which requires removal, at the mouth of the womb as this prevents the spermatic fluid to get inside and have the desired effect.

Barren Cow

Barren cows are very troublesome. It is best to keep them separate, as they often worry other cows and spoil them. So a barren cow should be carefully watched during these months, for if she calves once she may turn over a new leaf and take to calving again regularly. If a cow does not get into calf a year from the time she stops milking, or two years from the time she last calved, it is no use keeping her any longer; the probabilities are that she will never calve again.

Very often when a cow loses her calf, the *gowallas* resort to the wicked practice of *phooka* to extract her milk; apart from its being a cruel and inhuman practice, a cow that has once been subjected to it will never again have a calf, her generative organs having been destroyed or injured.

Great care should be taken to select a good bull to serve the cow. A good bull of a good milking breed will generally have calves of good milking strain. This is a subject to which special attention should be paid. If the cow is served, by a good bull it will not only ensure the production of a well-bred calf, but will also increase the quantity of the cow's milk and improve the cow.

It is not advisable to advocate English bulls for Indian cows. The pure-bred Montgomery, Sind, Hissar, or Nellore bull will prove the best. A cross-bred bull between an Ayrshire or Shorthorn cow and a Montgomery, Sind, Hissar, or Nellore bull will prove satisfactory.

It is a great mistake to send cows out to inferior bulls. The cowman, if not watched, will put the cow to the first bull which is at hand, which may not be at all a good animal. If a good and large cow be served by a small and inferior bull, generally the serving proves unproductive. On the other hand, if a cow has been troublesome about getting into calf, if she be sent to a large and good bull she generally conceives.

As a rule, cow-calves take after their fathers, and bull-calves after their mothers, but this rule is not is absolute.

Putting the Cow to the Bull

The most natural way is to allow the bull and cow to please themselves, and so leave them alone in an enclosure; but when a cow is restless, it is best to tie her up to a tree between two posts and secure her so as to prevent her from jumping about, so that the bull may easily serve her and not be tired out in attempting to do so. When a cow or heifer has been served, she should be tied up and left undisturbed; she will generally sit down quietly and not move for hours. It is best not to give her anything but some green grass or straw and water that day and subsequently for a few days more, and she should also be kept on low diet without any oilcake. A little soaked *kutheela* gum should be given her, and she should be bathed.

Heifers are sometimes troublesome on account of their timidity; and may not get into calf till long after they are old enough, and have to be put to the bull many times before he succeeds in covering them. They should be tied up so as to enable the bull to serve properly.

Chapter 18

Barren Cows

Because a cow has taken the bull and not become pregnant it is no proof that she is barren. Some cows, and especially the large well-bred ones, take the bull several times before they get into calf. A Hansi cow was served five times without any satisfactory results, but the sixth time she became pregnant. Sometimes cows give much trouble and annoyance and cause much loss of time, but perseverance wins the day.

If a cow has not got into calf within two years from the time she had her last calf, and is becoming fat, she is barren, and in all probability will never calve again. It is no use whatever keeping a barren cow.

Causes of Sterility

Over-feeding, or feeding on very heating food, will cause barrenness. Want of regular and sufficient exercise will cause the cow to become barren. Forcing supplies of milk by unnatural means will make a cow barren. Displacement of the womb, caused by accidents bad delivery or slinking, will cause sterility. Some organic or constitutional diseases, *e.g.*, leucorrhoea, cyst or other affections of the ovary will prevent conception.

It is said, if a barren cow is allowed to remain in the herd, others in that herd will soon become barren. The disorder is infectious, especially if it has been caused by a miscarriage.

Remedy

When a cow gives trouble about getting into calf, she should be considerably reduced in condition she should have only green grass, hay, and dry straw to eat. This treatment alone may cure her; she should be kept loose and made to take lots of exercise. If she still continues to give trouble, give her five to ten grains of borax every day, for five or six days. If this does no good, give her liq. ext. damiana 1 dram twice daily with food or water for a week. After the cow has been served she should be kept away at a distance from the bull and other cows.

Barrenness in Dairy Cattle

Many dairy farmers know, only too well, what it is to suffer great pecuniary loss owing to the barrenness of their cattle. The causes of this state of affairs are various and numerous, but among them may be enumerated the following:

Too high feeding may cause barrenness by causing the animal to become excessively fat, which interferes with the process of reproduction in several ways.

The remedy in this case is obvious, namely, to bring the animals down to a more reasonable degree of fatness.

Another cause of barrenness, and one which is equally condemnable, is that of keeping an animal in too poor condition. In such a case the animal can only just manage to keep afloat in the struggle for existence, getting enough food to satisfy the maintenance requirements of her mere body, but not enough to warrant her carrying on the important process of reproduction. The cure for this again is obvious, namely, that of getting the animal up to a better condition.

The keeping of an animal in a half-starved state deserves strong condemnation, and a farmer should, for the sake of his pocket, if not for that of his animal, keep his cattle up to a certain degree of fatness.

Barrenness, especially in highly-bred stock, may also be caused by too close breeding, i.e., by breeding from animals too closely related to one another. Close breeding is the best method to adopt in the formation of new breeds, but, carried too far, eventually results in a ruined constitution and weakened frame. Line breeding or, in other words, breeding from animals from one common stock, but not closely related, is the safest and most advisable method for the average farmer to adopt.

Sugar and sugary foods in general have a detrimental effect upon the reproductive organs of an animal, and therefore such foods as treacle, sweetmeats, etc., should never be fed in very large quantities.

The best foods to promote constitutional vigour are those containing plenty of phosphates, and, of course, a reasonable amount, but not an excess, of proteins.

Some animals are constitutionally barren, and nothing can be done to remedy this; while others may only have some small defect which is easily curable by a simple operation. Now that artificial insemination is so successfully practised, no valuable animal should be declared incurable until a Veterinary Surgeon has had a good look at her.

Old age may be the cause of sterility in older and in this case the only remedy is the weeding out of such animals from the herd and replacing them by younger and more desirable stock.

Sometimes the mouth of the uterus becomes very hard and the opening is blocked which makes a cow to be non-productive. In such a case the remedy lies in clearing up the passage by finger or application of some irritants, *e.g.*, red iodide of mercury ointment (1 to 25) by a Veterinary Surgeon and oral administration of ext. damiana liq. 1 dram for some days if the cow does not come to proper heat.

Another cause of barrenness, and one which seems fairly widespread, is that due to the action of a micro-organism living along the urino-genital tract and which, by causing the canal to become acid, destroys the vitality of the male sperm, and so producing barrenness.

An animal suffering from this form of sterility shows upon parting the lips of the vulva, a slight rash. This eruption is due to the presence of the micro-organism which causes the sterility. This form of barrenness seems to often occur when a herd is just getting over the effects of contagious abortion.

The best cure in this instance is the injection of a solution of potassium bicarbonate, one ounce dissolved in one pint of lukewarm water, and injected about one hour before the animal is served. This may, or may not, cause the animal to become pregnant.

Finally, in some instances the cause of the barrenness may be the fault of the bull. Some bulls have great difficulty to procreate a calf at all, while others will bred on one animal and not on another. In this case advisability of sending the cow to another bull discarding the old-one should be most carefully considered.

Chapter 19

Age of Cattle and Names at Different Ages

Age

The age of cattle is generally calculated by the growth of the permanent teeth, and also by the rings that form round the horns; but it is only after the third year that the circle on the horns becomes defined; so in calculating age by the rings, allowance should be made for three years; when an animal has six rings, it is eight year old (*see* plates). Of the two systems, that of judging by the teeth is by far the more reliable. At six years of age the eight permanent teeth are complete and attain a uniform level, and the mouth is said to be complete, literally what the Indians call *poora* in Hindi, and *pooro* or *poorno* in Bengali, when the animal has attained its prime. After this, the animal is supposed to decline or approach the age when its value decreases. After the sixth year nothing can be affirmed decidedly. Those, however, who have extensive experience with cattle can tell the age even after the sixth year with tolerable correctness. Careful examination of the teeth and of the extent to which they have been worn down, the marks (rings) on the horns-but the dealers invariably scrape them in order to avoid detection of the real age- and the general appearance of the animal itself frequently helf to determine the question.

At birth there are two central milk teeth, or incisors in the lower jaw, the upper continuing bare. During the second week after birth, four teeth make their appearance; in the third week, six; and when

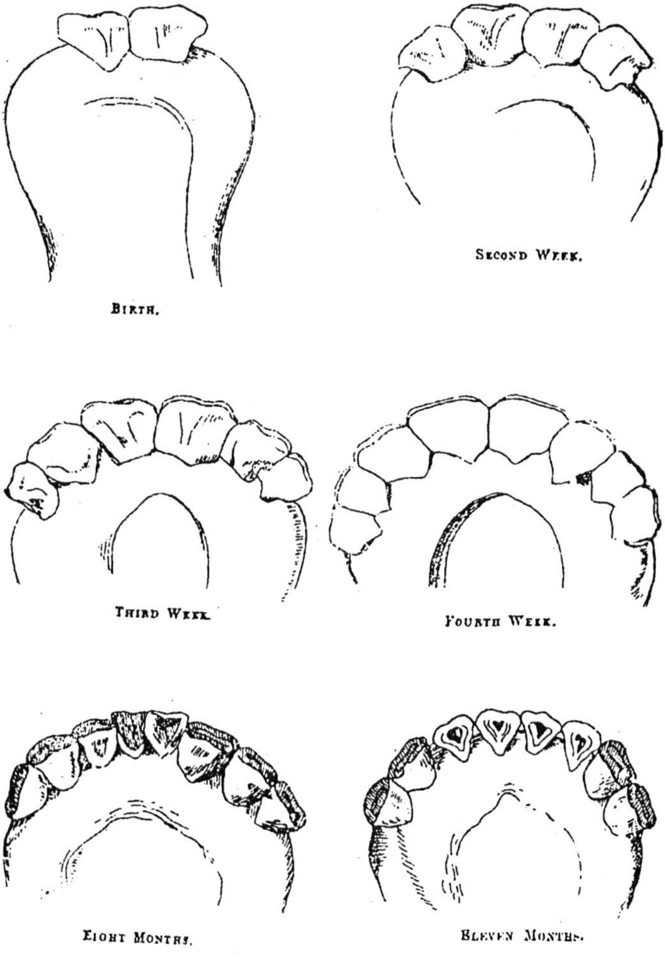

Fig. 40-45. Teeth at Different Ages

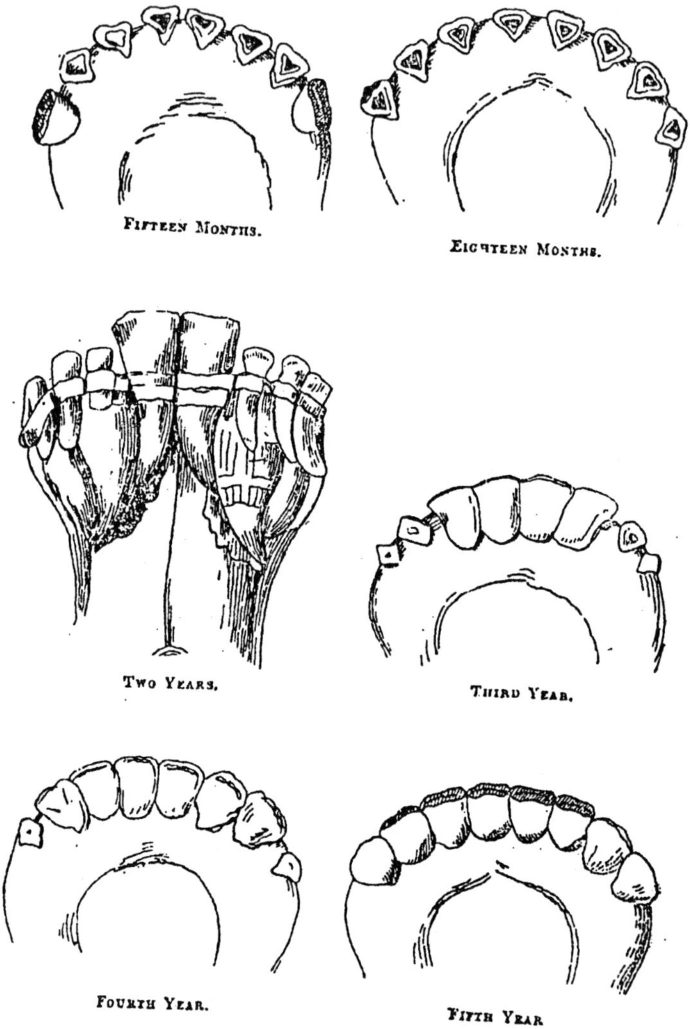

Fig. 46-51. Teeth at Different Ages

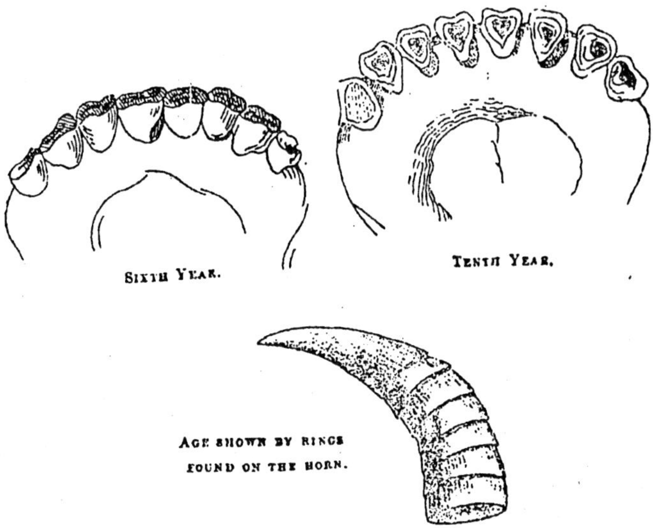

Fig. 52-54. Age Shown by Horns

the month has been completed, eight milk teeth have been established. Until the sixth month these teeth keep clean and even, but after the sixth month they begin to get discoloured and to wear down. The two central incisors first begin to wear down at eight months; four at twelve months; six at fifteen months; the whole of the eight teeth are well worn at two years, when also two of the central incisors are shed and replaced by permanent teeth, which are readily distinguished by their size and form from the milk teeth. At three years, four teeth; at four years, six, and at five years, the whole eight permanent teeth appear, and complete the mouth as stated above. At six years of age these in their turn will begin to wear down. But the extent of the wear of the teeth depends in a great measure on the kind of food the animal has been having. Cattle-bulls, bullocks and cows-attain to a good age when taken care of, and the reproducing powers of bulls and cows are retained for a long period.

The heifer breeds when she is from 2½ to 3½ years old, and continues to do so until she is twenty years of age; the bull is used for breeding purposes when he is three years old, and renders his best services until he is eight years old. After that he should not be used for breeding but put to the plough or cart. Sometimes he is used before he is three years old, but this is ruinous; if he be left until he is three years of age it will repay in the offspring.

Names of Cattle at Different Ages

The names given to cattle are as follows:

A new-born animal is termed "a calf," the male "a bull-calf," and the female "a quey," "cow-calf," or "heifer"; a gelded animal is called a "stot-calf." When a calf is a year old it is called "a yearling." When a heifer bears a calf, she is called "a cow," which name she retains ever after. A bull when castrated is called "a steer" until he is three years old when he is styled "an ox" or "bullock," which name is never changed.

A heifer or cow that has received the bull is said to have been served or covered. A cow that has not conceived or that has miscarried her young is an "eil," and one that has ceased milking is called a "yeld cow," or "dry cow." When in milk, a cow is termed a "milk" or "milch cow."

Indian Names

A calf is called a "butchroo" in Hindi, and a "bachoor" in Bengali. A bull-calf is a "sharh-butchroo" in Hindi, and "sharh-bachoor" in Bengali. A cow-calf is a "buckun" in Hindi, and a "bokkna," in Bengali. A stot-calf is a "budhia butchroo" in Hindi and a "bollod bachoor" in Bengali, and a steer a "bial" in Hindi, and a "bollod" or "damrah" in Bengali. A cow is a "gai," and a bull a "sharh" (nasal *sh*) in both Hindi and Bengali.

Chapter 20

Price of Cattle

The prices of cattle vary a great deal in different parts of the country, and at different seasons of the year. Cattle, in their own districts, are comparatively cheap, but the farther they are removed from home the greater their price. Prices of good cows, bullocks and bulls have considerably advanced during the past twenty years. In fact it is difficult to get really good stock now for even large prices, except from some of the Government breeding farms.

In Bengal from May to the end of September the fields are all under cultivation, and there is not much fodder for the cattle, consequently during these months they suffer from starvation and disease. Some of the ryots sell their cattle at this season, and buy again in October and November. The prices go up in October and continue good till the end of February. Some ryots, again, sell their cattle during the rains to enable them to pay their land rents. From October to December they reap their crops and are flush with cash, so they can again buy cattle.

Prices of Cows

The prices of cows are lower in their own districts and the farther they are taken from their homes the higher their prices. The prices of cows vary according to their breed and the quantity and quality of the milk they give. In Kolkata the standard price of a good cow in full milk, with a calf under a fortnight old, is as follows: If a large well-bred animal, at the rate of Rs. 25 to Rs. 30 per *seer* for every *seer* of milk she gives in twenty-four hours; if a medium-sized well-bred cow, Rs. 20 to Rs. 25 per *seer* for every *seer* of milk she gives in twenty-four hours; and if a small cow, at the rate of from Rs. 15 to Rs. 18 per *seer*. Thus a large cow giving ten seers of milk a day will fetch Rs. 250 to Rs. 300 and a small one giving less than five *seers* a day Rs. 75 to

Rs. 100. Some large well-bred cows sell at the rate of Rs. 25 to Rs. 30 per *seer* for the milk they yield in twenty-four hours. Sometimes when people are leaving the place and cannot take their cattle with them, they will sell them far below the standard price. Cows can also be got cheap at auction sales, but the buyer has to take risks in so doing.

In the Mofussil the prices of indigenous cows in milk are very much below the prices of the same animals in cities and towns. The cows that sell for Rs. 250 each in Kolkata can be bought for Rs. 100 or Rs. 125 in their own districts. *A cow is at her best value when she is between three and five years old, or with her second calf.*

By large pure-bred cows is meant cows of the Montgomery, Sind, Hansi, Nellore and Gir breeds; and by medium, good cross-breds; and by small, good common cows of the district.

When cows run dry, their value of course decreases; they can then be bought for from one-fourth to half or less the price of cows in full milk.

Prices of Bulls

The prices of good bulls are very high; one has to pay a big price for a fine well-bred bull. A good large pure bred animal when three years old will sell for from Rs. 200 to Rs. 400. A good Hissar stud bull has sold for Rs. 800. Good bull-calves of pure Montgomery, Sind, Hissar, and Ongole cattle can be bought for Rs. 60 to Rs. 100 when a year old; and from one to two hundred when between one and three years old.

Prices of Bullocks

The prices of good bullocks are also high. Good plough bullocks will fetch as much as Rs. 100 or Rs. 175 per pair. The common ones sell for from Rs. 50 to Rs. 100 per pair. Good cart bullocks will bring as much as Rs. 200 to Rs. 350 or more per pair. First-class pure bred animals will sell for as high as Rs. 300 to Rs. 600 per pair.

Breed, age, size, and strength make a great difference in the value of the animal. A bullock is at his best value when he is between three and five years old.

Prices of Calves

See Chapter 14.

Chapter 21

Milk

The quantity of milk obtainable varies considerably according to the breed of the cow, the kind of food she gets and the period of lactation. A pedigreed well-cared-for cow will give much more milk than a common one or a badly-cared-for good one. Some cows have given as much as thirty-six pounds of milk a day, but if a cow gives from twenty to twenty-eight pounds she is a good one. The season and frequency with which a good cow is milked also affects the quantity. When a heavy milker is milked three times a day she will give more milk than when she is milked twice; but when milked twice a day the secretion is believed by some to be richer and contains more butter-fat than when milked oftener. Climate also affects the yield of milk; too much heat, cold and damp are objectionable. A rich, dry soil is very favourable.

Cow that are stall-fed give more milk than those that are kept on grazing all the day.

A cow gives more and richer milk after her second calf than she did with her first, and it generally continues to increase until the fifth calf. When she is eight years old, that is, after fifth calving, her milk usually begins to decrease in quantity, but not always in quality.

Quality of Milk

The milk of every cow differs in consistency, quality, and colour. (1) There is the yellowish, creamy milk. (2) Then there is the thick heavy white milk. In good milk there should be at least four ounces of curd, and one ounce of butter to every pound of milk. The quality of food will also affect the quality of milk.

While the calf is very young the milk will be thin, but will get richer as the calf grows older. As a cow goes out of milk, the butter obtained from her milk will not lessen as rapidly as the milk itself does; the smaller quantity of milk will on account of its richness give a larger proportion of butter, and sometimes even when nearly dry a respectable quantity of butter will be yielded.

The milk of a cow immediately after calving is not fit for use it contains colostrum corpuscles. An hour or two after the cow has calved she ought to be milked and the milk thrown away; after this the calf should be allowed to suck the mother and drink all it can suck. Until the third day the calf should be allowed to suck all it can and the milk left must be drawn out and may be used for butter, *but should never be given to children.* After the third day the milk may be used for puddings and butter. After the tenth day the milk may be used for tea and coffee, *but is not fit for children to drink until the twenty-first day from the birth of the calf.*

The Lactometer alone cannot be relied upon as giving any absolute standard of purity. The solids of milk are heavier than water, but the fat (butter) is lighter, and very rich milk may rank lower, as shown by the Lactometer test, than milk that is really poor in quality (butter-fat). If sugar is added to watered milk, the Lactometer test will show it as pure milk. Then, again, by the Lactometer test the pure freshly drawn warm milk will rank as watered milk. The *gowallas* know this, and are up to the trick of making milk up to the Lactometer test.

Duration of Milk

Opinions differ as to the length of time a cow gives milk; some say a cow should milk up to a month of her next calving, but such a cow is rarely met with. Cows are in full milk for three or four months on an average: from the fourth month they begin to lessen by small degrees, during the seventh month there will be a decided decrease; they go on milking for two, three, or four, and even seven months longer, but by this time the milk will have almost dried up. Some cows keep up the full supply of milk for six months and more, and then gradually decrease and do not stop altogether until their calves are twelve to fifteen months old.

Some cows calve every year or thirteen months, and only milk for eight or nine months. Do not stop milking a cow until three months before the time for her to calve again. A cow if allowed to go dry early will do so again the next year, whether she calves early or not. But it is a "penny-wise pound-foolish" principle to keep on milking a cow until two months of her time to calve again. She is given three months' rest, as a rule.

When a cow is going off her milk, any change of food, quarters, attendants, time of milking, or the man who milks her, etc., will often accelerate the decrease and she may not recover herself, and the milk may stop altogether.

When a cow seems to be going off her milk, apparently without cause, it may be that she is out of sorts, and that her digestion is out of order; in such a case an ounce of the condition powder made into a drink with treacle and water, and given for a few days, will often restore her appetite, and give her digestion the required tone. The calf should be let loose for a day or two; its continual sucking may bring back the milk which has been checked.

Papeeta (Papaya) leaves and green fruit will often bring back a flow of milk if it has stopped from any disorder in the cow's health. The leaves and fruit should be pounded together, and mixed with a little flour and treacle and given in balls or mashes.

The Art of Milking

A cow should always be fed before she is milked. Few can milk a cow without first allowing the calf to suck the teats, and the cow seeing the calf near, allows the milk to flow; sometimes it will be seen that both udder and milk increase rapidly in the space of a few minutes. The cow will then relieve herself as Nature dictates, and when she has done so, her calf should be tied to a peg near her head, or to her foreleg, where she can lick and fondle it while she is being milked. A kicking cow should be shackled, but not a good-tempered one, as it is a bad habit to get them into, and may induce them to kick.

The cow should always be milked by the same man for a change of milkers may make her nervous and affect the flow of milk; cows like being milked if the operator has a gentle touch. They are creatures of habit, loving peace and quiet and regular routine; if they are always fed at the same hour, and milked at the same hour, in the same place and by the same man, they will seldom rebel.

If a cow is troublesome at milking, the milker should be changed; a good man will always have his cows quite docile, and though one may be ticklish and difficult to milk when first put under his care, in a short time he will have her quiet and patient.

Sometimes a cows teats get chapped or inflamed, and she kicks about to let her distress be known. Chapped teats are most troublesome, and with some cows they are constitutional, but as a rule they are the result of leaving the teats wet after milking, and allowing them to dry in the open air. To avoid this, the cows udder should be well cared for, and, from the very first, butter or a mixture of six ounces of any bland oil and two ounces of spirit of camphor should be rubbed in. It is well to rub some butter or ointment over the teats for a month after calving, as then they harden without chapping. Chapped of teats are very painful and may cause the cows milk to dry up.

If the calf nips its mother with its teeth, it must not be allowed to suck her too long at a time.

Young Cows Need Careful Milkers

Many young cows are absolutely ruined by careless or rough milkers during the first weeks of the milking period. Through bad treatment they get a bad reputation as poor milkers, while the fault lies entirely with those who handle them. A good milker is probably a greater rarity than a good cow, the cow is a sensitive creature and requires to be handled in a gentle manner. No portion of her body is more sensitive than her udder. It is a great relief to the cow to have her distended udder relieved of the milk there is in it, but she expects it to be drawn quickly and gently, no unnecessary tugging at the teats, but by a gentle, rapid pressure, and with a downward movement of the fingers.

As a rule, with her first calf, the cow's udder is swollen and tender, and the skin is very sensitive. It is wise to wash the bag and teats with soap and warm water and wipe dry, and apply bland oil after milking. With clean cows and clean cowsheds, the next step should be a clean milker, and to be a clean milker does not necessarily mean that a man must wear a white duck suit. It does mean that he must have clean hands (with finger nails cut short and washed with soap and water), clean clothes and clean habits.

The Process of Milking

The milking of a cow is a very simple process when one is used to it but to do it successfully and correctly, without causing pain or annoyance to the animal, is the secret, and requires skill and experience. Milking may be performed in two ways, by stripping or nievelling. Stripping consists in seizing the teat at its base with the forefinger and the thumb; and drawing them down to the end of the teat, pressing it lightly so as to bring away the milk it contains. Nievelling, as it is called, is effected by grasping the teat with the hand and compressing it against the palm with the fingers to drive the milk out, and then relaxing the hold to allow the teat to refill, so that, by a quick succession of contraction and relaxation by the hands, the milk is soon drawn out from the udder; only large cows with large teats can be nievelled; small cows can be milked only by stripping. Every milkman prefers his own method of milking, and it is no unusual thing to see a man use both stripping and nievelling on the same cow in the course of one single operation; habit has a great deal to do with the practice. The milking should be done quickly, the longer the milker takes in extracting the milk the more restless the cow becomes, and the quantity of milk yielded is affected. A good milker will extract all the milk in half the time that an inexperienced man will take.

The Milking Utensil may be an earthen bellmetal or brass *lota*, galvanized bucket, tin can, or enamelled pot. Whatever the utensil may be made of, it must be kept absolutely clean and sterile with boiling water and soda but copper utensils should never be used for milking.

When the Calf Dies, there is usually great trouble in milking the cow. As soon as the calf dies endeavour should be made to give the cow another calf of the same age, colour, and sex as her own calf. It is to be seen that the calf is quite healthy and clean, and then about a couple of ounces of milk newly drawn from the cow, should be rubbed over the head face, back, and upon the genital organs of the calf. The cow will smell and lick the calf, and soon allow it to suck her. Some cows will take to another calf, whereas others will not. When she will not take to another, her dead calf has to be skinned and stuffed and stuck up before her for her to look at and lick while the milking goes on. Unless this be done she will not let her milk down; but even with this device her milk will gradually lessen, as the average milker will not be able to extract every drop. As soon as the calf dies, a *mochee* or tanner should be sent for, the calf skinned, and the skin cured and stuffed and dried in the sun. Only salt and lime to be used on the skin, and *no* arsenic. If the calf has died of any contagious disease, its skin will carry the contagion, so it should not be kept.

Every Drop of Milk Must be Extracted from the cow both morning and evening. After the milker has drawn away all he can, the calf must be let loose and allowed to suck so that every drop may be extracted; any milk left in the udder tends to dry up the cow, as what is left becomes absorbed and the flow of milk is lessened. The more the cow is milked and the more the calf sucks, especially during the first three weeks, the more milk will be produced.

Great care must be taken not to, in any way, annoy or startle the cow before or during milking; any rough treatment will make her restive, and she will not allow herself to be milked. Servants need to be watched carefully, for very few will obey in this matter .

Cows Holding Up Milk

It is quite common to find cows that have the bad habit of holding up their milk–a thing that is hard to overcome unless a person knows just how to go about it, There is always a definite reason for it however, as a cow that has everything to please her physically and mentally will be very unlikely to hold up her milk, and when a cow that holds up her milk is put in physical and mental comfort she will quite probably give it down again. *Farm and Home* (England) discusses this subject briefly in a way that gives some interesting points to dairymen, and says: "Cows are often 'difficult' in regard to giving down their milk perfectly in the height of the milking season. They fall into the habit in the flush of feed from tenderness of the udder, especially if the time between milkings are unequal, so that at one of them the bag becomes very much over-strained and painful. The bag thus becomes inflamed, swollen, and hard, and withholding the milk or any part of it tends to increase the difficulty. From an unequal division of time between milking, some cows habitually hold up their milk at night and give it down in the morning. The habit once being formed there is no sure cure for it. The same treatment will not work alike on different cows. As a rule, cows give down best in a few minutes after they first come into the stable or yard without having any food before them or anything to attract attention or disturb them, but some will give their milk more freely if eating something that they relish well, so that their attention is more taken up with the food than the milking. Regular, evenly timed, quick, quiet and comfortable milking is essential, and the best means both for preventing and for breaking up the bad habit in cows of holding up their milk."

Forcing Supplies of Milk

Some people give cows large drinks of hot water with bran, flour, or sugar sifted into it to make it tasty, so that they may drink largely and give a larger supply of milk. Others again give large quantities of salt to the cows to produce thirst, so that they may drink water to excess. Some resort to the diabolical practice of *phooka*, in order to extract milk. The least that can be said about these unnatural means resorted to by some unprincipled people, is that they are highly injurious to the cow, and invariably spoil the milk. Milk produced by such methods becomes watery and is unwholesome, as it does not contain all the nourishments in the shape of vitamins. Again, this forced increase is always followed by a reaction, and the supply of milk lessens considerably. Besides all these, it is most injurious to the cow. It affects her digestion, and causes much internal distress, and destroys her reproductive powers, so that she may never calve again. This is how large numbers of good cows in dairies and cities are ruined for breeding and future dairy use.

Fig. 55: Milk Tube

Importance of Regularity in Milking

In everything regularity is a good practice, but in good dairying it is imperative. To produce large and rich yields of milk is the sole function of the dairy cow, and to do this she must be of good dairy type, fed on palatable and nutritious foods and milked clean at regular periods. Dairy cows are rightly said to be milk producing machines turning concentrates and roughages they take, into milk.

As a rule the cow is milked at 5 o'clock in the morning in summer and 6 or 7 o'clock in the morning in winter; and in the evening at sunset. Two very unequal periods are made for the cow by this sun-to-sun milking, and as a consequence the quality of her milk flow and the length of her annual period are reduced. The cow can do her best only when milked at equal and regular daily periods of about 12 hours apart the year around.

The full supply of milk is not in the udder ready to be drawn out before milking time comes, but two-thirds of it is produced by the glands during the operation of milking. The udder, however, is usually filled and the cow becomes accustomed to this, but if the milking is delayed and the udder becomes unusually full, it begins to pain the cow and the glands cease to some extent to secrete more milk, and they will then not be stimulated to good activity during the process of milking. This injures the glands and produces a decrease in the milk flow. So it is very important that the milking be done regularly at as near the same time each morning and evening as possible. And it is also well that persons doing the milking do not change, for each one has a little different manner of milking than another, and a change causes the cow to feel uneasy, and in some cases if the change is repeated too often, it may injure the udder, and the cow will give less milk.

At milking time it is best that the cow be comfortable and contented; she should have consumed at least a portion of her feed before the milking begins, so she will have been satisfied and willing to part with all her milk. It is also well that clean, fresh water be offered her before milking.

The job of milking cows is probably a drudgery to more milkers than a pleasure. Conditions in the dairy easily become such that the work of milking is dreaded. The man who doesn't try to enjoy his work usually allows such conditions to obtain, and the more he dreads the work the worse the conditions, and vice versa.

With cleanly conditions, convenient facilities for feeding and caring for the cows, and gentle cows (indicating kind treatment), the task of milking can be made quite as agreeable as any other work upon the farm. That is, providing the milking is not done when one ought to be in bed, and, providing, further, that he really takes pleasure in this kind of work.

Chapter 22

Cream

Watered Milk

Milk that has been watered always looks bluish, which can be detected by looking at a little in a wineglass; it appears more transparent than pure milk. Highly adulterated milk can be detected by taste also. Watered milk has a wholly different flavour and feel to the tongue: it is harsh and tasteless, while pure milk is soft, sweet and smooth. The glass bulb or Lactometer for testing milk is not to be wholly relied on. The milk of an old cow is rich in butter-fat than the milk of a young cow. The different kinds of food given to cows will affect the specific gravity of their milk as well as butter-fat.

Milk that has been watered will not turn sour sooner than pure milk. If milk turns sour sooner than it ought to do, one may suspect its being not cleanly handled. Another way to test the milk is to let it stand for a short time and a cream line will be formed and seen if kept in a transparent glass receptacle; if the cream comes in a thick crust, it is pure; if it breaks up on skimming and will not readily come off the milk, it has been watered, and the skimmed milk will then be of a bluish colour, and look like white agate or opal. It is difficult to skim watered milk, but pure milk is easily skimmed, as the cream is thick and solid.

Cream that has been skimmed off the milk that has been properly boiled and allowed to stand sufficiently long, makes good butter. Indians make another kind of cream which they call *kheer* or *khoa*. It is made by simply boiling down the milk to a very thick consistency. This cream is not suitable for making butter or ghee but is largely used for making sweets.

Keeping Milk Good

Milk will keep good if a few points are carefully observed. China crockery retains heat and may turn milk sour if retained for a long time. The best kind of vessels to keep milk in are aluminium pans, from twelve to eighteen inches in length, seven to nine inches wide and one-and-a-half to two inches deep.

They should be well scrubbed with dry wood ashes and soda until every particle of grease is removed, washed with cold water then scalded with boiling-water, dried with a clean piece of linen and put in the sun to dry.

These pans should be placed side by side on a shelf and filled three-fourths with milk. The milk should be kept in a quiet room which is not used as a passage, and which can be shut up and kept cool. If people come in and out of the room they will disturb the atmosphere, and prevent the cream from properly forming. When the weather is warm, the doors of the room should be opened out at night. The atmosphere of the room should be cool and the pans placed on cold water if possible.

The milk vessel must not be moved or touched from the time it has been set to the moment of skimming.

Cold is favourable to the forming of cream; some people place their milk vessels in wet sand.

Changes in the weather affect milk very much; sometimes on a cloudy day the cream will be quite thin, and a fall in the barometer will soon sour the milk; milk and cream will lessen when a westerly wind blows; frost will prevent cream forming; a bright, clear, and calm day is most favourable. The wind can be shut out by closing the doors and windows. Should the milk turn sour any day, one need not be discouraged, as it may be a storm is brewing and the electricity in the air has turned the milk, or else the pan is dirty; when things go wrong, the cause to be looked for and if possible to be removed.

Skimmed Milk that has stood not longer than twelve hours is good, and may be used for all household purposes. If reboiled, skimmed milk will keep good for many hours; when milk has stood for more than twelve hours, it should not be used for the table, but it will make good curd, or may be given to ducks, fowls, dogs, goats, and other; animals. Skimmed milk, pure and undiluted, also contains a great deal of nourishment, and, as it is cheaper than pure unskimmed milk, should enter largely into man's daily food.

Boiling Milk

In the hot weather and rains milk will not keep good for any length of time unless it is properly boiled. Boiled milk produces proportionately more cream than unboiled milk does. Milk intended for cream and butter should be boiled for a longer time than milk used for tea, coffee, and for children.

Susceptibility of Milk

Milk, cream, and butter all take the flavour of any strong odour which may be near or about them. Milk while it is being boiled is sometimes turned sour if it be old and stale.

Iron turns it red and makes cream black.

Copper vessels, unless well tinned, should not be used for storing or boiling milk; brass turns it green and gives it a nasty flavour. When kept long in iron vessel, milk turns blue when put into tea. New earthen pots give milk, cream, and butter a strong and unpleasant earthy taste.

China is a retainer of heat, so that all milk jugs, cups, and basins are unsuited for keeping milk in for a long time.

Aluminium, zinc, bell-metal, and wood are also utilised as milk vessels.

Milk is a favourable medium for the growth of microorganisms, and being easily infected usually carries infection to the unconscious consumer. If milk is bought from the village or bazaar, it should be thoroughly boiled before using, or else it is certain that one may be infected with any disease prevailing in the bazaar or village.

Separators for extracting cream from fresh milk are now used largely by dairymen. Cream so extracted is called "fresh cream" and is used for tea, coffee and puddings, and for making butter. The separated milk is most wholesome and, if thoroughly boiled, may be used for all household purposes and making curd.

Chapter 13

Butter

Boiled and Unboiled Milk

Until the thermometer rises to 70° butter may be made from cream of unboiled milk.

Butter is usually made from cream separated from raw or boiled milk by ordinary cream separators procurable from the market, the prices of which vary from Rs. 90 to Rs. 350. For thorough skimming the temperature of the milk should be about 100°F. when it is put in the separator. The cream thus collected is kept for about 24 hours to ripen, when it is churned in a butter churner by diluting the cream with icy cold water to bring it down to a thin consistency and at a temperature of about 58°F. Cream obtained from raw milk can be pasteurized by placing the vessel containing it in boiling water, till the temperature of the cream rises to 145°F. and then holding it at that temperature for half an hour and subsequent cooling.

Butter thus made has, as some think, a finer flavour than butter made from cream of boiled milk; but boiled milk yields more cream and butter than unboiled milk does.

If all the milk is. used for butter, then set it for twenty-four hours; the cream then, will collect into a thick paste, leaving the milk below quite thin and poor, unfit for household use, but good for fowls, ducks, goats, dogs, etc. It will also make curds.

If the milk is to be used for butter as well as household purposes, it should not be allowed to stand for more than twelve hours in the cold weather, and an hour or two less in the hot weather.

It is more profitable to make butter from cream, and to let the milk stand for only twelve hours, as then the whole of the milk can be used for the household, and also a sufficient quantity of butter produced. Skimmed milk should be reboiled thoroughly.

If the milk stands longer, there will be more cream and butter, but the milk will be useless.

If there be more milk than is needed, then the surplus can be sold after it has been skimmed; skimmed milk will sell for from two to three pice per pound.

Collecting Cream

When the cream is skimmed, collect it all in a large mug or bowl until there is a large quantity. Stir the whole with a fork every day. When two or three days' cream has been collected, the butter may be made. But by keeping the cream from twenty-four to forty-eight hours it ripens and thereby helps in churning.

The process of butter making is exceedingly simple. Butter made from cream must be made in a Dazey or some such churn. These churns can be had at all hardware shops.

Butter made from sour milk or tyer is best made ill the indigenous churn in the popular way. It will not yield much butter in a Dazey churn.

The indigenous churn and mode of making butter are both very simple. This method of making butter produces a lesser quantity of butter than when prepared by churning cream obtained by a cream separator. Another objection is that all the milk is lost, as the whole of the milk turns sour. This sour butter-milk cannot be used for puddings, tea, etc., but, when fresh, it makes a very refreshing and nice drink, and is very cooling in he hot weather. It is liked very much by Indians and some Europeans. It is also very good for dogs and poultry, and when in large quantity, some curd can be had out of it.

The milk is boiled well, after which it is put into a large jar, and a teaspoonful or tablespoonful of sour butter-milk or tyer is added to it, and it is put aside for twenty-four hours, when a quantity of *cold* water is added to it, and it is churned. From one to one-and-a-half ounce of butter is produced from each pound of milk, if made by this method.

The churning apparatus consists of a stake some four feet long driven into the ground; to this, two feet art from each other, are tied two rings made of cane bamboo stick. The jar containing the milk is placed at the foot of the stake under the rings, and the churn is passed through the two rings into the jar. Then a string put round the churn between the two rings, and the urn is drilled for twenty minutes.

The churn is simply a piece of thin, smooth bamboo, five feet long, split into four at one end, and opened out to the width of three or four inches with small pieces of bamboo placed crosswise to keep it open; this end is placed in the milk, and the churn is drilled.

The butter forms and floats in the jar, when it is collected, washed in cold water and salted. Nearly all cooks and people know how to make butter in this way.

The butter-milk will sell for from one to two pice a pound. Many people drink it, and also give it to their pigs, ducks, fowls and dogs.

When boiled, sour butter-milk turns into curd. The water should be drained off and the curd washed with warm water, then pressed and used for the table.

Dazey Churn

This is the best churn for use of small households. By making butter in the Dazey churn, you save nearly all the milk, though the quantity of butter is not great. By the Indian mode of making butter one can get from one to one-and-a-half ounce of butter from every pound of milk; by making butter in the Dazey churn with cream, one gets only from half to three-fourths of an ounce of butter from the same quantity of milk, but the whole of the milk, is good for use.

All the cream should be put into the churn, and a little *cold* water added. The water cools the cream and helps in churning. Commence churning slowly and if the temperature is not sufficiently low add some broken ice to the cream and continue; the more slowly the butter comes, the better it will be in both quality and quantity.

The churn must be securely closed. Care should be taken that the man does not hold the churn with his feet, or it will make it warm and make the butter oily.

As soon as the fluid becomes heavy and cloggy, the churning should be done more slowly, and continued so until the churn runs easily again, and the sound of the fluid rattling about inside be distinguished; then the churner should look to see if grains of butter are forming, and continue churning gently until the butter forms solid lumps in the churn.

If the butter is turned out before it has formed solid lumps a great deal is lost, as it is impossible to collect all the small particles when it has once been taken out of the churn. Servants, if not watched, will always take it out too soon.

When the butter is ready, pour off the butter-milk and give it to goats, dogs and fowls. Wash the butter with *cold* water which has been standing all night in an earthen *sorie* or *ghurra;* in case ice is not procurable fresh water from the well or tank or tap is sure to be warm, and will melt the butter. After washing the butter thoroughly, it should be salted and made into pats, and put into an earthen pot filled with *cold* water. Butter made in this way will keep sweet and nice for many days.

Butter should never be touched with the hand or left in a warm place for even a few minutes. A wooden or bamboo spoon and knife should be used. The churning should always be done early in the morning.

After the thermometer reaches 70°, butter-making becomes troublesome, as the heat makes it soft and oily. Pieces of ice should be dropped into the churn while churning to harden the butter, and the churn should be placed in a tub of cold water.

Cleanliness

Want of perfect cleanliness is a great obstacle to successful butter-making, especially so in the hot weather; and without the eye of the housekeeper perfect cleanliness is not to be obtained as most of the servants do not seem to realize the benefits of cleanliness. Neglect of this may spoil the whole of the butter. The same spoon that has been used to skim the morning' milk should not be used to skim the evening's milk. All the vessels and implements should be kept perfectly clean, and soaked in clean water until the time they are needed for use. Deal and bamboo are the only kinds of wood that should be used in butter-making.

Preserving Butter

After churning, wash and salt the butter, and keep it in an earthen (*mutti*) vessel full of cold water in a cool place; the water must be changed morning and evening. The ice-box or refrigerator, etc., are good place to keep butter in.

Sweet or Sour Cream

"Sweet cream is not the best for making butter, as it yields less than cream that is slightly sour. The best and most butter is made from cream that is slightly sour, and which is taken from milk set in shallow pans in a room not over sixty or sixty-two degrees of temperature for thirty-six hours, then skimmed and kept twenty-four hours at the same temperature before churning and churned at this same temperature. When cream is too sour or is too warm, it will foam in the churn and give out a large quantity of carbonic acid gas. This interferes with the making of the butter. It will not do this otherwise. To bring the cream, when thus disturbed, into proper condition, add cold water to thin it, by which the gas evolved in the churning escapes and the foaming is reduced. Then the butter separates. This foaming is a common thing in the summer, while in the winter, owing to the cold, the cream granulates and appears to be sandy and the butter does not come. The remedy then is to add warm water to the cream, as it is too cold, and the fine grains of butter will not adhere together."–*American Farmer.*

Chapter 24

Ghee

Making Ghee

Collect all your spare butter of the last few days, and put it into a small aluminium pan on a clear charcoal fire, or oilstove, slow fire (*not too hot*), and let it boil gently. Always have it done in your presence in some convenient spot. At first it will froth up like whipped cream, then by degrees it will curdle, and small white opaque particles will be observed inside; after a time the particles will begin to collect to the bottom of the pan, leaving the *ghee* quite clear; when it is nearly ready it will leave off frothing and will simmer quietly, rising in round glossy bubbies; now stir gently with a spoon, so that the froth at the top may go down, but do not disturb what has caked at the bottom, which after a time will look like a poached egg; while all above will look like salad oil, clear and bright. It is now done. Take it off the fire, strain through a piece of fine cloth and pour it gently into an empty bottle with a large mouth, and, when cool, cork down tightly and cover the cork with bees-wax, sealing-wax, or bladder which has been soaked in bluestone and water, otherwise the ants will eat off the cork and bladder.

As the *ghee* cools, it will look like good honey. If carefully made it will keep good for some time.

The great secret in making *ghee* is patience. It must not be boiled on too hot a fire, or it will burn, turn brown and smell nasty. To make ghee from salted butter is difficult and requires experience as it goes on frothing even after it is ready to be taken off the fire and does not burn and gives off nasty smell.

Home-made *ghee* when used for cooking is just as nice and wholesome as the best butter, but the bazaar *ghee* is nasty adulterated stuff.

Clarifying Ghee

If *ghee* has been kept any time, and there is a doubt about its sweetness, or if *ghee* has been bought from the bazaar or village, it should be turned into a saucepan, and re-boiled. Put a cupful of milk, with a few cloves and lemon leaves into it before putting it on the fire. By adopting this process a nice flavour and colour can be given to it.

Chapter 25

Curd, Cheese and Tyer

Curd is a very useful article of food, and makes many delicious dishes, *e.g.*, varieties of sweetmeats for the table. It enters very largely into the diet of the people of India, and in some places during some seasons of the year sells as high as 1½ to 2 pounds for the rupee.

Making Curd

Curd is made from fresh milk, separated milk, or skimmed milk. Sometimes skimmed milk several hours old, turns in the boiling of itself, if put on fire; but fresh milk will not curdle if put on fire immediately or after few hours unless some acid is added to it.

Put the milk into a saucepan, and put it over the fire; let it boil up, then put a dessert spoonful of butter into it and stir well, or put a cupful of whey, or half a cupful of sour butter-milk or tyer, or a little lemon juice, and keep stirring. In a little while the curd will form and separate from the whey.

If fine soft curd is wanted, then drain off the whey while it is hot and use the curd immediately.

But if large-grained hard curd is required, then let it cool before draining off the whey; put it in a piece of clean cloth, tie tightly, and hang it up and let the last drop of whey drain off. This will give one a nice cake of curd. Unskimmed milk produces better curd than skimmed milk does. Curd made from skimmed milk is tasteless and cannot be sold to the public as it falls under the Food Adulteration Act.

Cream Cheese

Cream cheese is best when made from curds of fresh unboiled milk. The process of making it is very simple. Turn the milk, put the curds into a clean cloth, and let the whey drain off. Open the cloth, remove the curd, place it in a plate or dish, add salt to taste and thoroughly mix; then put it into, a clean cloth, carefully fold the cloth over it, and place it on a piece of board under a good weight till the remaining whey is drained off. When this is done it is ready for use. Cream cheese is very good when fresh, but it will not be nearly as nice if kept long. When making cheese from skimmed milk some cream should be added to the curd and properly mixed.

Tyer

The Indian name for tyer is *duhhee*. It is made thus–Take two or three pounds of pure, fresh milk, boil for some minutes and to facilitate cooling pour it into a large-mouthed shallow dish; an earthen (*mutti*) *handi* (especially made for the purpose) is preferable. When it is lukewarm, *i.e.*, about 107°F., dip a teaspoon containing just a little quantity of 12 hours old tyer in the middle of the milk and place it in a quiet warm corner preferably on wooden planks and cover the *handis* up with a blanket, and let it stand for twelve hours, when it will be ready for use.

Chapter 26

Lice, Ticks, Flies etc.

Lice

Cattle must be kept perfectly free from all kinds of vermin. When their coats are long, especially in the winter, cattle are troubled much by lice of a bluish colour and very small. If these are not immediately removed, the cow will get quite sickly from the great irritation. The insects are so small that they will escape detection unless the coat is carefully examined. When one observes a cow rubbing herself constantly, he should look for parasites.

Calves often get them in large numbers, and of neglected become very weak and die.

The cure is simple: Rub phenyle and water, or some of the liniment mentioned at the end of this chapter, well over the animal. Apply the remedy for three days and then bathe with any toilet soap in warm water. Do this for two or three weeks.

Dog-ticks also attack cows. Ticks must be carefully picked off. They cling about the udder, and under the elbows of the poor creatures, in places where they can neither be scratched nor rubbed off, and a cow will often put down her head and sigh with relief when they are removed.

After the ticks have been removed some naphthalin balls (powdered) or some of the liniment should be rubbed over the animal.

"Flit" or a like stuff may be conveniently sprayed both for as a preventive and curative over the tick-affected parts or the whole body.

Flies trouble cattle very much. The gadfly bites very severely, also the common house-fly will get in under the hair of the cow and worry her. If cattle are properly groomed and kept thoroughly clean, and be occasionally washed with a weak solution of phenyl, they will not be troubled very much with flies.

Mosquitoes also plague cattle very much. The cattle house must be properly smoked every evening. Burn some refuse straw and dried cow-dung at the door of the house windward on a slow fire. This will drive the mosquitoes away.

Throw a little incense on the fire.

The following application is a good cure for lice, ticks, etc.:

Cocoanut Oil	10 ounces
Kerosene Oil	4 ounces
P. Camphor	2 ounces

Heat the cocoanut oil and mix the camphor and when cool add kerosene oil and keep in a bottle well corked. Mix well and rub over the animal. Care must be taken not to allow the stuff to get into the eyes or licked by the calf.

Another good remedy is to rub *neem* oil on the affected animal, and after three days bathe it in warm water with any toilet soap. Do this twice a week for a couple of weeks.

Chapter 27

The Seasons of the Year

It may be said that in India the year is divided into three seasons-the cold, the hot, and the rains.

The cold weather usually lasts from the 15th of October to the 1st of March. At this season the cattle need more nourishing food, and a greater quantity of it, than in the hot weather. At night they should be always covered with a blanket or a warm coat called *jhule* especially made for them, or else kept in a warm house.

Keeping cattle out of doors in the sun during the day except from 12 to 2 at this season, does them good, but they must be protected from the cold draught and rain, and always be placed in a warm house during the night. The milch cow feels the cold very much, and her milk is very much affected by it.

There will be sufficient grass on properly managed lands for the cattle at this season. From the end of September to the beginning of March, a good stock of hay, *bhoosa* (chaff), and straw must be stored up for the cattle to feed on from the 1st of March to the 15th of July, when grass and straw will be scarce. If this is not done, the cattle will suffer and become diseased. From October to March one can get grain and chaff cheap, and it is advisable to buy then and store away for use during the year. In February wheat, kullie, and other chaff can be obtained in abundance.

The hot weather begins from the 1st of March, and ends by the 15th of June to the 1st of July. At this season cattle suffer much from want of food, and, if not cared for, will naturally get reduced and may even die; but they will keep in better condition on the same quantity that they got in the cold weather. The midday sun is injurious, but all cattle may be tied out of doors at night with advantage. A close stall will lessen the milk of a cow.

At this season there will not be any green food for the cattle, and they must be given an abundant supply of hay, *bhoosa* (chaff) and straw during the day and at night.

Tender green leaves also are very good for them. It is best to grow some special green food, *e.g.*, Guinea-grass, etc., for the cattle at this season.

The rains begin from the 15th of June to the 1st of July, and end by the 15th of October.

At this season there is an abundant supply of grass and other green food for the cattle.

Cattle will not suffer any ill from drizzles or light showers of rain; but great care must be taken that they are not exposed to heavy rains and storms or put into their stalls at night while they are wet. Servants must be constantly watched, otherwise they will leave the cow-house dirty and wet, and this will be very injurious to the cattle.

Cattle should never be tied out at night during this season, and should be carefully protected from all storms and cold winds.

Cattle may be let out during the day at all seasons, and they will not suffer any inconvenience, if only they are protected from the midday sun, storms, heavy rains, cold cutting winds and damp. They must not be allowed to graze on marshy grounds, or lands that are not properly drained.

Great care must be exercised at all seasons to guard the cattle against contagion. The farther they are kept from the public roads and the village cattle, the better.

Chapter 28

Cattle-Dung

Cattle-dung is largely used by Indians as fuel in towns and cities. The villagers utilize this also for manure as well as for plastering their mud houses. It is mainly used for manuring their lands; for better harvests. The commoner classes of Indians who have cows but own no land, never buy wood or coal for fuel; they make dung cakes or rolls, and dry them, and cook their food with them. Often they have more than they need for their own use, so they sell the surplus to those who require them.

Profit

The dung, when it is fresh, can be sold or made into cakes or rolls for fuel, or it can be turned, into manure and sold. A properly fed cow will produce at least a pice worth of dung every day.

Manure-pits

For making manure, a pit six feet square or larger, according to the number of cattle, and six feet deep, should be dug, and all the dung and refuse foods thrown into it every morning and evening. When, the pit is nearly full, a lot of water should be poured over the heap to make the stuff moist, and then it should be covered over with a foot and a half or two feet of dry earth. The pit must be kept closed for six months; after that the manure will be fit for use in the fields.

These pits should be a good distance away from the dwelling-houses and cow-sheds, and not only far from but below the water-level of the tank or well. Great care must be taken to properly cover the pits; any negligence in this matter may cause much sickness and loss.

Chapter 29

Grazing Fields

Providing fodder for cattle in India is a subject deserving the most serious and careful consideration of all ryots and zemindars, and the Government.

There is a great necessity for pasture-lands as without this cattle can not thrive well in any country. The cattle are left to browse on the roadsides, or are tied near their house to only gaze at the fields of paddy and wheat around them. No special grazing field is provided for them. The consequence is that the cattle are only skin and bones, and so weak and stunted that they are unable to do much work. Besides, a great number die every year, and the ryots are unable to cultivate their lands. The result is, the people are not able to pay their rents, or have sufficient food for their families. Every village should be compelled to have grass-lands for its cattle.

The chief cause of the present bad condition of the cattle and the scarcity of milk and ghee in the country is partly due to the scarcity of grazing fields.

In certain sections of the Punjab, United Provinces, and Mumbai and Madras Presidencies, certain tribes and people breed good cattle and take good care of them and grow fodder, and so some good cattle are found at those places.

There should be a law compelling the zemindars and ryots to reserve land in every village for grazing cattle. One and a half *biggah* per head of cattle should be the minimum allowed. If there be 200 heads of cattle in a village, there should be 300 *biggahs* of grazing and reserved in this village. Each cattle owner should be compelled to reserve one and a half times as many *biggahs* of land for grazing as the number of cattle he has. The zemindar should take not more than four annas a year per *biggah* rent for this land, and the cattle owner should be punished if he uses it for any purpose other than grazing cattle and raising fodder for his own cattle. The District Board or Local Board of the district should select the land to be thus reserved in each village. This could easily be decided at a conference with the Agricultural Veterinary officers and the people of the district.

Some Europeans and Indians of the richer class buy fodder for their cattle, and do not let them starve or suffer. But buying grass and green food is very expensive and the poorer people cannot do it.

If one have a piece of land that he can set apart for his cattle, he will do wisely if he cultivated fodder. It will be cheaper to grow it than buy it, and his cows will be sure to have green food all the year round.

Amount of Land Needed

Three and a half *biggahs* or one acre of land will be sufficient to provide green food for one cow the whole year round. For village cattle even one and a half *biggah* per head will suffice to keep them alive, but good cows cannot thrive on less than three and a half *biggahs*. In dairy-farms, where the cows consume large quantities of food, it will require two acres or seven *biggahs* to supply a cow with all the grain and grass she needs. (A Bengal *biggah* is 14,400 square feet, or 120 feet by 120 feet).

Some say it is best to grow grain on the land and stall-feed the cattle. Others again say it is more profitable to grow only grass and hay, for then the cattle will have a greater abundance of food and will thrive better. It is advisable that, of the seven *biggahs*, three ought to be left in grass, and on the remaining four *biggahs*, barley, kullie, wheat, *joar* and special fodder grass should be grown. This will give the animal sufficient grass, grain, chaff, hay and bran during the year.

Fertility of the Land

Pasture-lands need proper management. Many persons graze their cattle on the land from January to December, or cut away the grass and never think of doing anything to improve the lands. They think grass-lands need no care or management; but this is a serious mistake. The very best land could not long bear this strain upon its productive powers.

There are two ways of retaining the fertility of land; either by the application of manure, or by stirring up of the soil. Proper and regular irrigation is necessary for improving the grass-land. In some parts of India there is to be found some water which runs to waste but could be turned to account during the hot weather, for the improvement of the grass-land, if only a little ingenuity were exercised. But in most places water is very scarce in the hot weather, and it would be a great expense to irrigate the land. Lands on the banks of rivers, or between two rivers, are very suitable for grazing and raising fodder; and cattle do best on such ground if it is properly drained. The best and easiest method is to manure the land every year.

The best time to manure the land is from March to the end of May, when the land is almost bare; the early showers will speedily wash it down to the roots of the grass.

Preparation of Land

Before the manure is put down on the ground all the jungle and coarse patches of grass must be taken up by the roots. The enormous; strain made upon the land by all this jungle and coarse grass renders their extermination necessary. After this, the land should be well ploughed and harrowed, then the manure should be put over the land, and the plough and harrow drawn over it again, and the stones picked up. After the harrowing, the land should be properly levelled and rolled. The ploughing is necessary only for the first manuring; the second year the land should be well weeded and rolled, and the manure put down, and the harrow passed over it; after this, the stones should be picked up. Or else the manure can be put on the land in trenches nine inches deep and then covered over with three inches of earth. If this is done the land will need neither ploughing nor manuring for five years. If the manure is not put in trenches the land should be ploughed thoroughly every year or second year. The trenches should be from 25 feet to 30 feet long, 10 feet wide, and 9 inches deep. Such trenches should be made on the whole of the land, and the trenches filled to three inches of the surface with all the refuse, droppings and sweepings of the cow-sheds, stables, gardens, poultry and sheep yards, and with night-soil. Each trench when filled should be covered over with three inches of earth. The grass on this land will be better the second and third year than the first.

Draining

Grass-lands must be properly levelled and drained, and should the drains become faulty, they must be repaired. Unless the lands are well drained, the grass will be stunted and coarse.

If the lands are properly manured and drained, there should be an abundant supply of grass the greater part of the year; and if irrigated, the whole year round.

Doob is the best grass to grow. If one finds the grass on the land is coarse and of an unnutritious kind, *e.g.*, "*uloo*" then it is necessary to thoroughly plough up the whole land, break up the earth, remove the roots of the coarse grass and weeds and manure well, and sow the *doob*. The *doob* is very nice and soft, and very nutritious, and all animals eat it very greedily. The seed of the *doob* can be obtained from any of the gardens. If the seed is not obtainable, it is advisable to take up a lot of the grass by the root, and to cut it up into pieces (one inch long), and to scatter it over the land, and put the harrow over it. Guinea-grass is also very good for cattle.

Lucerne grass, or clover in large quantities is bad for cows in India, as it is very heating and dries up the milk and makes the animal want to calve long before the ordinary time. It may be given to bulls, bullocks and horses, and also to young heifers if one wants them to calve early; but as it tells on the cow's constitution if she calves when too young, and the calf is likely to be weakly, it is better not to hurry nature. Not more than from two to four pounds may be given a day, and then mixed with other grass. If one can afford it may also be given to troublesome dry cows in order to bring them into season early.

Green Food

Wheat, barley, kullie or woorid, Indian-corn, *joar*, bujri, shama, ground-nut, when they are green and tender, make splendid food for cattle and make the cow's milk very rich and nutritious.

Sorghum Poison at Different Stages of Growth

It has been known for some years that sorghum and similar plants, grown in rich soils, were more liable to contain dangerous amounts of hydrocyanic acid-commonly known as "prussic acid"- than when grown in soils poor in nitrogen. It was found that the nature of different soils very largely governed the amount of those poisonous properties in the plant.

Determining the stages in the growth of sorghum, when the poison in it would be at the danger point, was a very interesting and valuable phase of the investigation. It was found by experiments that sorghum grown in highly rich, nitrogenous soils could not be freely fed to animals with safety until the plant is preparing to seed.

The sorghum plant grown under the conditions described-when very young, and from the age of 3 up to 7 weeks-contains distinctly dangerous amounts of prussic acid. After that age the poison rapidly disappears by decomposition, the nitrogen passing over into other and strictly nutritious elements of food. When the flowering stage is reached, not more than a trace of the poison is found–*Extract from Agricultural Journal of India for April 1902.*

Chapter 30

Dairy-Farming

Dairy-Farming

It is often said that it is impossible for anybody in this country to make a living by dairy-farming; and it is said of several persons who have sunk large sums of money in the attempt. On inquiry it has been found that these persons failed because they had no knowledge whatever of the business, and went about the whole thing in a way that certainly could not ensure success. Some people seem to think all they have to do to work a dairy is to buy a few cows and employ some *gowallas* to feed and milk the cows and sell the milk. They know nothing about cows, so they get their servants to buy them; they know nothing about feeding cattle, so they allow their servants to give the cows whatever they please; they know nothing about the care of cattle, so the cows are not cared for properly; they also know nothing about milk and butter-making, so these things are entrusted to the servants, and the milk and butter may contain anything. These people start with a great noise and flourish, and induce some of their friends and neighbours to patronize them; but in a short time they are unable to supply what they agreed to supply, and what they do supply is of doubtful quality; so in a little while their customers, one after another, withdraw and go back to *gowallas,* or try to find a more reliable source of supply. The cost of servants and food for the cows exceeds the receipts for milk and butter produced, and the poor dairyman finds himself in debt, if not bankrupt, and in six months or a year the business is closed. This is the disastrous experience of most people who have tried to do this business in this country. Now, anyone with any sense will see that people of this type will never succeed in dairy-farming.

There are certain things necessary in dairy-farming and without these essentials it is impossible for anyone to succeed in the business. First, the person--be it man or woman-must have some practical knowledge of the business. That is, he must serve an apprenticeship of at least one year in some properly conducted large dairy before he can work one himself. Second, he must be diligent and prepared to do a large portion of the work himself. He must known what to do and when and how to do it, and must order and supervise every detail of the work personally, and not allow any servants to manage or interfere with the business. The servants must be under his absolute control. Third, he must be absolutely honest, and not allow any of his servants to do anything that he himself would not do. He must do all he can to merit the confidence the people have placed in him in taking his milk and butter. Fourth, he must be able to supply the demand for milk and butter as the demand daily increases. If, even for a short time, he is unable to do so, the people whom he has failed to supply will seek other sources for their supply, and he will probably lose their patronage permanently.

As has been said above, the four things essential to dairy-farming are-knowledge, diligence, honesty, and capital: without these four combined no one can possibly succeed for any length of time.

Dairy-farming has a much more comprehensive meaning in India than in Europe. The duties of a dairy farmer in India are multifarious, and he must be familiar not only with all branches of the dairy industry but also with the allied subjects. The requirements and qualifications of a dairy farmer are well summed up in the *Journal of Dairying*, Vol. I, No. 1 (October 1913):

"A dairy farmer must be:

1st: A good business man, or he cannot make his, farm a financial success.

2nd: A keen observer, as his business is made up of innumerable details, which must be seen to by him personally.

3rd: A hard worker, as he must always be engaged in his work, for he is never finished; it therefore follows that his recreation must be found in his work.

4th: A good breeder, as his success depends on his being able to get '*two cows under one hide.*'

5th: A student and investigator–the first, as he must keep up his study to keep in touch with new methods; the second, as he must introduce new ideas to suit his particular environment.

6th: Well trained in practice and theory–theory to guide him in a correct practical method.

7th: Trained to absorb new methods, as these become necessary; and he must know the best grasses, crops, weeds, also all poisonous plants.

8th: An intensive farmer, as he must use his manure and raise heavy crops continuously for green feeding on his own land.

9th: The chemistry of feeding-stuffs, soils, manures, and dairy products should be studied to show him the, cycle of application. (For balancing the rations-S.N.S.)

10th: The elements of bacteriology studied, to show him the need of cleanliness, so that harmful bacteria shall not influence the quality of his produce and its keeping powers; and what pasteurization and sterilization mean.

11th: A mechanical training is necessary to enable him to keep his machinery in order and prevent its failure, what machinery is necessary and which is the best for his purpose.

12th: A knowledge of heat is required to enable him to know the principles on which his refrigerator works, and his cold store is kept cold.

13th: A veterinarian, to enable him to keep his cattle in health and to treat them when sick."

India is Certainly One of the Best Countries for Dairy-Farming

Land and food-stuff are comparatively cheap, labour is cheap, cattle are cheap, and the milk of the Indian cow is just as rich as the richest milk produced in England and America. Most of the cows in India are equal to the Jersey cow for richness of milk. Then, again, milk and butter bring higher prices in many places in India than in England and America.

A few figures here will be interesting. In England it takes from two and a half to three and a half gallons, or twenty-five to thirty-three pounds, of milk to make one pound of butter. In India it takes from fourteen to twenty pounds of milk to make one pound of butter. In England good butter fetches from one shilling to one shilling and two pence a pound; in America the same butter will sell for from twelve to twenty-two cents a pound; and in India it will bring from one rupee to one rupee and twelve annas a pound. Then, again in England fresh milk sells for from eight pence to one shilling a gallon; in America such milk will fetch from twelve to twenty cents a gallon; and in India one will get from one rupee to a rupee and twelve annas for a gallon of pure fresh milk.

It costs less to produce milk and butter in India than it does in either England or America, and milk and butter sell for higher prices in India than they do, under normal condition, either in England, Australia, or America. Now, if the above-mentioned facts prove anything, they prove that it is quite possible to successfully work a dairy-farm in India.

Experience

It is advisable for any person wishing to start a dairy-farm to first spend a year in one of the first class dairy-farms in India, or in one of the Government Military or Agricultural dairies, and study every detail of the work. Some small private dairies can be conducted successfully by studying books and buying knowledge from daily experience, but for dairy-farming on a large scale a practical knowledge of the business is absolutely necessary to start with.

Capital

To make a dairy-farm pay enough to enable a man to comfortably support a family, it must be worked on a large scale. From fifty to a hundred cows must be kept. The outlay for cattle, lands, buildings, utensils, implements, etc., will be between thirty and forty thousand rupees. A dairy with twenty cows will cost between fifteen and twenty thousand rupees. The outlay could be considerably reduced by renting lands and houses instead of buying and building. But the high rents will take away a great deal from the profits. Small dairies with three or four cows can be successfully carried on to supplement the family income.

The Position of the Dairy-Farm

The dairy should be situated in the suburbs of a city or town, or near a city or town, close to a railway station. The milk and butter must be delivered at regular hours to the consumers; the usual times are between five and six o'clock in the morning and four and five o'clock in the evening and unless the dairy is so situated that this can be done conveniently and at a small cost, it will be impossible to conduct the business successfully.

The position of the dairy must be elevated above the surrounding land, so as to give a natural drainage. The ground must be perfectly dry, and even during the heaviest rain no water must lodge on any part of it. Attached to the farm building, or immediately adjoining it, there should be a large tract of land for grazing dry cows and calves, and for letting out milch cows for exercise. There should be two acres or seven *biggahs* of land for each cow. A dairy with one hundred cows will need two hundred acres of land. If it is impossible to obtain all this immediately near the farm building, there must be sufficient land near it to enable the milch cows and little calves to exercise, and tne grazing lands may be situated farther away.

The land should be divided into different plots. About a third should be allowed the cattle for grazing and exercise, and two-thirds cultivated and sown under barley, wheat, kullie, *joar* and fodder grass for cattle food. There should be large trees on the land to give shade to the cattle. Good clean water should always be accessible to the cattle.

The Class of Cattle Needed

The success of a dairy depends in a large measure upon the cows in the dairy. If the cows are bad milkers, they will eat much and yield little. The dairyman must procure and produce the best milkers. By best milkers, is meant cows that will give the largest quantity of milk, containing the largest quantity of butter-fat. No cow giving less, than 3,600 lb. of milk, yielding 180 lb. of butter, in ten months, is worth keeping in a dairy. A cow that gives twenty-four pounds of milk and one and a quarter pound of butter a day is a good cow. Some cows will yield from twenty-four to thirty-two, pounds of milk a day and produce one and a half to two pounds of butter. Some cows will milk for ten or twelve months, others, again, will yield only for six or eight months. It is always more profitable to have the best. It is a "penny-wise and pound-foolish" policy to buy cheap cows that will yield little milk, and that only six or eight months.

Greatest emphasis is laid on the point that a dairyman should select his cattle with the greatest care, for his success or failure will depend much upon these cattle. Good cows will be found among every breed; some crossbred cows are very good milkers. By crossbreds, is meant crosses between pure Montgomery, Sind, Hissar, Nellore, Gir, or English cattle, and not between the better breeds and the common village cattle. It would be advisable for dairymen to select their cows from among the following pure breeds–Montgomery, Sind, Gir, Hissar, Nellore, or crosses between the English cow and bulls of the above-mentioned pure Indian breeds.

The Montgomery and Sind cows produce the largest percentage of butter-fat. Some of them have given as much as 7 percent. This is equal to the best Jersey cow's production, and as good as the majority of buffaloes will do. It costs much less to produce milk and butter from a Montgomery and Sind cow than from a buffalo, who eats so much more.

Dry Cows

It will always be found more satisfactory to keep the best cows after they become dry than to sell them. If the cows are properly managed, they will milk for three or four months after calving, and then take the bull. They will continue to give milk for six months after taking the bull, then remain dry three months, when they will come into the dairy again in perfect condition. This subject has been dealt with more fully in a previous chapter.

Breeding for the Dairy

It is more profitable for a dairyman to breed his own cows than to buy them. If the dairy is properly managed, and there are good grass-lands, this can easily be done at a small cost. (*See the chapter on Breeding*).

Bulls

Every dairy should have a couple of really first-class Montgomery, Sind, Hissar or Nellore bulls to serve the cows as they come into season. Unless this is done, the cows will become permanently spoiled. (*See previous chapter on this subject*).

Important Matters

There is some evidence to the effect that in the Civil Dairy, Poona, and in other dairies, good cattle bought outside tend to deteriorate in the subsequent lactations under the conditions that are found in a large dairy farm, and that their progeny also tend to deteriorate. This is the case both with cows and with buffaloes. It is admitted that the milk value of the bulls used in such dairies is little known, but presumably the bulls used are as good as those in villages, and the fact that the original animals purchased deteriorate in subsequent lactations indicates that the defect is not in the breeding as carried on at these dairies. The feeding is undoubtedly better than is usually found in villages, and the housing more sanitary. This falling off can therefore be attributed to defective tending. It is probable that in any country the small owner who treats his milk animal as "one of the family" will always get better results from it than the large dairy farmer, with whom the animal is merely "a business proposition"; but the men usually available for employment in Indian dairies have, as a rule, little knowledge of cattle and they are frequently bad milkers and careless tenders. This constitutes a serious difficulty. It has already been written about the mode of feeding cattle, the need of exercise, cleanliness, regularity, kindness to the cows and calves, rearing calves, etc., and it will be referred the reader to those chapters for information.

The "Journal of Dairying" says–Live stock should be carefully and judiciously selected to suit the locality. The three best breeds of Indian cows are undoubtedly the Saniwal, Sind, and Hansi. The first is most suitable for the Punjab, the second for Scind and the Mumbai Presidency generally, the last named for the United and Central Provinces.

"At the present time it is really difficult to get reliable bulls, so that the improvement of these breeds is very difficult."

"It has been found necessary to import good bulls from Europe where large quantities of milk are necessary, but it is a risky proceeding, as the latter are subject to the trying heat and all the infectious diseases of the country. It is, therefore, the duty of every well-wisher the industry to strive for an improved type of indigenous cattle."

"It is absolutely essential that dairy farmers rear the young of the most profitable animals and thereby work up a good herd of home-bred stock, gradually increasing the minimum yield per annum until it high standard is obtained. Cattle giving less than 3,000 lb. per annum are not usually profitable.

"Good feeding with succulent crops or silage, a grain or concentrated ration of sufficient food value to maintain the cattle in good condition and to accord with the milk yield is important. The dry and young stock must also be kept in the pink of condition if the herd is to be improved."

"The rearing of calves is a matter of great importance. A calf that is not well reared can never be expected to become a good breeder or yielder. The first weeks of a calf's life are the most critical."

"Considerable improvement is often possible in many dairy herds, because, although an average yield of 5,000 lb. per annum is regarded as satisfactory in this country, yet it is by no means uncommon for individuals to give eight or nine thousand; these figures are therefore obtainable."

"The first step to take in improving a herd is to inagurate milk records if they are not already in vogue. The farmer can then select with exactness the heifer calves from his deepest milkers for subsequent retention in the herd. Though it is not definitely certain, there is, nevertheless, every probability that the progeny of a deep milking cow will also develop deep milking qualities. It is, however, more necessary that the maternal ancestors of the bull used in the herd should have been deep milkers."

"Cows also require careful management, or the effect will soon be seen in a diminished milk yield. Their milk-producing organs should be well developed by careful and thorough milking of the young cow, every drop of milk being stripped from her at each milking time."

"In the feeding of dairy cows, each individual animal should be studied, and rations given her which will keep her milk yield up to its highest pitch."

"The milk records will show the effects of different rations, and the cow's highest limit of quantity can soon be determined, beyond which any extra food is waste."

Profitable and Unprofitable Cows

Only a rich man can afford to keep inferior cows. Sometime, it is said that a man, unless he is well off, cannot afford to own good cows; but that is not true. If he can afford to own a cow at all, he can afford to own the best. The man who refuses to take the necessary steps to secure a good cow must work double time to get any profit, and wait years before he can breed up to a higher standard. It has to be realized at the beginning that it is better to put all the money in one or two good cows than in a dozen inferior ones. The profits of dairying depend entirely upon the cows and the system of raising food and giving it to the animals. It has been proved that good, not fancy-bred, cows have made good profit per year for their owners, after the cost of feed and all other charges had been deducted. If one good cow will make, that profit, a herd of 10 or 20 should net a fairly good income. This can be done in almost any region where good methods of farming and dairying are observed. More can be accomplished, but this is enough to show what some dairies can and are doing. It matters not so much of what breed they are, so long as the animals are adapted to dairying and are good representatives of their breed. Each animal must be judged on its individual merits, and if not up to the standard it should be discarded. Price does not always measure the value of the profitable cow. Sometimes high prices are tacked on for cattle of certain structural forms and breed–characteristics which would not be of any use to the ordinary dairy farmer.

Buffaloes

Most of the dairies in India keep large numbers of buffaloes for milk. The better bleeds of buffaloes give large quantities of milk; some have given from five to eight gallons, that is, fifty to eighty pounds a day. The milk is much richer than cow's milk. It usually takes ten to twelve pounds of this milk to make one pound of butter. Buffaloes are very large and gross eaters; they will consume three times the quantity of food a cow will consume and cost much more to feed. Buffaloes are more delicate than cows, and succumb to disease much more quickly. The buffalo-calf is more difficult to rear than the cow's calf.

Buffaloes are considered by many to be altogether unsuitable for dairy purposes, and the chief reasons for coming to this conclusion are, first, the milk of the buffalo is very heating and unfit for human consumption until it is first skimmed and largely diluted with water. It may prove less injurious in the hills and colder climates, but is absolutely harmful in the plains. Parents who have the welfare of their children at heart should never allow them to have buffalo-milk. If this milk is given to children, they will suffer from liver, bowel, and other complaints caused by biliousness and other stomach trouble. Mr. H.A. Howman in his report on dairy work in India, submitted to Government in 1890, fully corroborates the above statements. He says buffalo-milk is very likely to act prejudicially on the liver of both children and invalids. He found that buffalo-milk was used in the Scottish Orphanage at Mumbai, and this milk often made the children ill. Unscrupulous dairymen sell diluted buffalo-milk for cow's milk or mix the two together and send it out as pure cow's milk.

It is a most significant fact that experienced Indian horse-breeders will not give buffalo-milk to young horses, because, as they say, horses reared on buffalo-milk succumb to heat and fatigue much sooner than horses reared on cow's milk.

Indians make tyer and ghee from buffalo-milk, but very few, except the hill tribes and people of the colder parts of India, will drink the milk itself. Buffalo-milk is considered very much inferior to cow's milk, and if cow's milk sells at twelve pounds for the rupee, buffalo-milk ought to sell at sixteen pounds. In some places where milkmen buy up the milk in large quantities to mix with cow's milk for sale, or butter makers buy it for making butter, the price of buffalo-milk is higher than cow's milk.

Secondly, the butter made from buffalo-milk is not nearly as good as butter made from cow's milk. Buffalo-butter is very white, and has not the nice flavour of cow's butter. To remedy this, a lot of colouring and flavouring has to be used; but notwithstanding all the doctoring this butter has to undergo, it is very inferior to butter made from pure cow's milk. The only thing it is good for is ghee. If butter were made from unadulterated buffalo-milk and then turned into ghee, it would serve a useful purpose; but most of the buffalo-mill ghee sold in the bazar is adulterated with a stuff called "Vegetable Ghee" (vegetable product), and also with certain oils and fat. The better class of Indians have a strong objection to ghee made from buffalo-milk. If "Gowah ghee," that is ghee made from cow's milk, will sell at one pound for the rupee, "Bhainsha ghee"–ghee from buffalo-milk-will sell at one and a half pounds for the rupee.

No dairyman can afford to make ghee for sale. It will take about one and a quarter to one and a half pound of butter to make one pound of ghee, and ghee sells at a lower price than butter. The dairyman should let buffaloes alone, and confine his operations to cows only.

Some Difficulties

The dairyman must not think that all before him will be smooth sailing. He may by proper care and watchfulness keep disease away from his cattle; he may by proper selection and good management make his cows yield large profits; he may by fair dealing and punctuality gain a large constituency; but he will have to fight for the victory. The chief enemies are the servants. His own servants will lie, steal, neglect the cattle, shirk their duty, and give no end of trouble. He can never trust a single man so as to depend upon him absolutely. He must watch them closely, and stand over them in everything they do; otherwise they will soon defeat him and cause endless loss. The servants will be in league with the people outside. The man who supplies the oilcake, grain, chaff, or straw will find it to his advantage to give the servants a certain percentage on the amounts consumed, so that the consumption will increase; and it will be to the servants' advantage to run up the food-supply bills as much as possible, and if they cannot do this, they will steal the food-stuff and starve the cattle. It will be to the chamar's advantage to give the servants so much for each skin he can get, and the master will wonder why his cattle are dying never suspecting that the good servants have poisoned his cows and calves. It will also be to the advantage of the milkman (*gowala*) to get this dairy out of his way; so he takes the servants on the dairy-farm into his confidence and service to gain his purpose, and the dairyman will find his cows do not yield the milk or butter they should. Then, again, there are the servants of the consumers. They want, *dustoori* or bribes. If it is not given, the milk is tampered with and no end of complaints are received; and then, in a great many cases, the milk is rejected. Finally, there are the ignorant and senseless masters and mistresses who are controlled by their servants and will believe all and do all their mischievous servants tell them. These are the chief trials and difficulties in the way of the dairyman in this country. If he can surmount these, his success is assured.

That dairy-farms on a large scale can be conducted successfully in this country by Europeans and Indians is conclusively proved by Mr. Keventer's Dairy-farms at Aligarh, Simla, Delhi, and Kolkata, and Mr. Brown's "Express Dairy-farm" at Behala, Kolkata. These farms are conducted on right business principles and are properly managed and yield satisfactory profits. They have spared no money in providing all the necessary buildings and the best up-to-date appliances, and have a good staff of trained assistants. The initial outlay and the annual running expenses are large, but the profits have been large enough to cover all expenses and leave a substantial surplus.

There are still a number of so-called dairies conducted by Europeans, Indians and Anglo-Indians in Kolkata and other places in India. From what has been seen and learned about them it was very evident the proprietors knew nothing whatever about dairying on management of cattle. The whole business was conducted by and for the benefit of the *gowallas*, cattle dealers and butchers, who seemed to form a joint stock company, and sooner or later the owners had to seek the protection of the Insolvency Court.

Chapter 31

Breeding and Rearing Farms, Dry-Cow Farming and Cattle-Shows

There are three ways by which we can preserve and improve the best breeds of cattle in India.

Breeding Farms

First, by establishing breeding farms in parts of the country best adapted for the purpose. There are many places in India specially suited for cattle breeding.

All over India, in villages and bazaars, we find some small cultivators, traders and labourers–who are not *gowallas*–keeping one or two good cows, selling the milk and successfully rearing the calves. Such people should be encouraged as much as possible.

Then there are some people, especially in the Punjab and Mumbai and Chennai Presidencies, who breed larger numbers. A few of them do well, but most of them are not very careful in their methods and do not get the best results.

We have a few large and properly managed breeding farms established and worked by Government, such as in Hissar, the Lower Bari Doab Colony and Montgomery, and Military and Agricultural Dairy Farms in Allahabad, Lucknow, Lahore, Amballa, Ferozepore, Jubbulpore, Poona, Belgaum, Quetta, Sind, Pusa, Rungpore and in other places where very good cattle are bred. But these farms are not sufficient to supply all India. Such breeding farms should be multiplied in large numbers all over the country. This could easily be done by the many ruling princes, chiefs, large landlords, rich professional men and merchants in the country, for they are the inhabitants and permanent residents of India and if the best results are to be attained the process must be continued for many years, from generation to generation.

There should be some large farms and many small ones. The larger ones could be worked better on scientific lines and would be more successful and profitable. The smaller ones could be conducted by small landowners and large farms under the guidance of expert Government officers.

The cows, bulls, bullocks and calves from these breeding farms would always be sought for by the people and would fetch good prices. If cattle-breeding were properly organized and controlled, there would be, in a few years, marked improvement in cattle all over India. One thing must be insisted upon, that breeding operations must not be left in the hands of ignorant and superstitious people, who will not weed out the unfit and useless cattle, and will breed from stunted, decrepit and diseased ones. If breeding farms are to be a success, trained men must be placed in charge, and very strict selection of the breeding stock must be made. Only the best cows and bulls must be retained. If the best are retained, then the unfit and useless must be got rid of. If these rejected cattle were only used for slaughter instead of the good ones, it would be a great benefit to the country. For some years it may be necessary for Government to assume control of some of these farms, and when properly established hand them over to people of the country who are able to continue the work on the same lines.

All cows and heifers unfit for breeding purposes must be eliminated, and all bull calves not fit for breeding must be castrated.

Cattle-breeding could be made profitable if conducted along with dairy-farming by educated youths, planters, zemindars, retired civilians, military officers and others who have facilities for it.

Rearing Farms

The second way the best breeds of cattle could be preserved and improved is by establishing rearing farms in large numbers. Such farms could. be worked in many places more successfully than breeding farms. Young calves could be procured from good breeding and dairy-farms and reared until they are three years old and sold at a good profit.

A large number of cultivators, shop-keepers and labourers in many parts of India buy one or two young calves and rear them until the heifers calve and the bullocks are broken to the plough and cart, and then sell them at good prices. These calves are usually well cared for. The women and children of the house take a special interest in them, feed and tend them and treat them as members of the family. They bring grass for them, give them the leavings of the *dal* and rice when husked, vegetable pealings, all the rice water and some oilcake. Some of these calves grow up to be fine animals and fetch very good prices, but they are not always good specimens of pure breeds. If those people could be induced to select really good pure-bred calves, rearing them would be very much more profitable and a greater benefit to the country. These small rearers are important factors in the problem of cattle improvement in this country, and everything should be done to encourage them. There are many people who have very little land and no means of keeping breeding cattle, but they could very easily rear one or two good calves, and this would pay them better than growing paddy on a couple of *biggahs* of land.

We need these small rearers, but to improve the cattle on a large scale rearing must be done on a large scale. This part of agriculture could well be taken up by educated youths, the well-to-do classes who have lands that could be used for grazing and growing fodder. The most successful method would be to reserve large tracts of good grass-land and keep from fifty to one hundred head of young cattle. They will need to be stall-fed as well as grazed, as is done at the Hissar and other farms.

Young calves can be bought from the Military and Agricultural dairies or from private breeders and dairies when the calves are weaned. Some of these dairies sell some calves when a few days old for a nominal sum, but, calves from eight to twelve months old will cost from thirty to sixty rupees each. If these calves are properly reared they should fetch from Rs. 150 to Rs. 300 each when three years old.

Dry Cow Farming

The best way of saving good milch cows from being slaughtered is for people to start farms for keeping dry cows until they calve again. Some large farms could be established, and it would pay the proprietors very well. It would also pay people to keep three or four dry cows at a time.

One of the two following plans could be adopted to procure dry cows for these farms. First, private gentlemen and dairymen who have good cows that have run dry, whether in calf or not, and have no ground and conveniences for keeping them, should send them to one of these farms, or send them in ones and twos to people in the mofussil, and pay from five to eight rupees a month for the food and keep of each it cow until the calves again. After she has calved the owner will take the cow back and send another one in her place. In this way owners can save their good cows at the cost of Rs. 60 to Rs. 96 for each, and get them back in full milk. If the cow does not get into calf within twelve months from the time she calved before, she should be sold to the highest bidder.

The other plan advocated is for the owner of the farm to buy up all the good dry cows he can get from private parties or from dairymen and keep them until they calve again.

The *Jain* people have what are called *Pinjarapols* or *Gowsalas* all over the country. All sorts of cattle, good and bad, young and old, healthy and diseased, are gathered together in these places for the purpose of preventing their being slaughtered. The condition of some of these places and the cattle kept in them is very deplorable. Many of these *Pinjarapols* are really cheap dairies that get cows for nothing.

Many people have mistaken ideas, and send their dry cows to these places. These cows are lost to the country for all useful purposes. If these institutions were properly kept and the cows and calves properly fed and cared for, and when the cows calve if they were returned to their owners or sold to respectable people under certain conditions, there would be a great deal to be said in their favour. The calves should be sold to people who will rear them properly for agricultural purposes or for milk. If these institutions sold cows to European and Indian gentlemen at reasonable prices, or lent them on the condition that when the cows were not needed any more they would be returned to the institution, many good homes would be found for good milch cows, where they would receive better treatment than they receive in *Pinjarapols*.

Good milch cows of the Montgomery, Bind, Mooltan and Hissar breeds, when they stop milking, are sold by milkmen and others to butchers far from Rs. 30 to Rs. 80 each. If these cows were bought for such prices and sent to these farms or to private individuals in the mofussil where they would be properly kept and fed until they calved again, they would sell at full prices of cows in milk. If a cow is bought for Rs. 50 or Rs. 60 and kept twelve months, the cost for food and keep for the period would not be more than from Rs. 96 to Rs. 20. If the cow calves before twelve months, the cost would be proportionately less. When she calves, her price will be from Rs. 250 to Rs. 300. This would bring in a profit at the very least of Rs. 60 to Rs. 80 per cow.

But suppose one of the cows dies or is proved to be barren. Even in that case the loss would be less than the gain. The probabilities are that only one in every ten cows will prove barren. There is always a risk in buying a dry cow that one knows nothing about. She may be barren, caused by bad feeding, want of exercise or by the cruel practice of *phooka,* but a person with some knowledge and experience of cows or a Veterinary Surgeon can without much difficulty discover if the cow has been ruined.

If the calf died long before she ran dry she may have accumulated fat, or her udder may have been spoiled and her teats dried up, or she may have been subjected to *phooka* and had her generative organs destroyed. If her calf is alive, it is very probable she is all right and will calve again. If she is in calf, then there is no risk whatever if her teats are right. If the cow is still giving some milk, one can always tell in what condition her udder and teats are.

Because a cow has taken the bull two or three times and not got into calf, it is no proof that she will not calve again. If the cow is fat, she needs to be reduced in condition before having her covered.

There should be one or two bulls of the best milking strain in every farm for dry cows, and the cows must be covered as soon as they are in season. People who undertake to keep a few dry cows must procure a good bull, unless there is a good bull near-by that can be used for the cows. Even if there is a good bull in the neighbourhood, it would be advisable for a person to keep his own bull, for any delay in serving a cow will be a great loss of time and money.

Dry cows must have a lot of grazing. They cannot be kept profitably in confinement. They should be given an abundance of green grass, hay, or *bhoosa*. If she is fat, plenty of grass, straw, hay, *bhoosa* and water will be all she needs. If she is rather out of condition, she will need feeding up, and one or two pounds of gram should be given with cut grass. If she is in proper condition, she should be given two pounds of wheat-bran in the morning and two pounds in the evening with cut grass or *bhoosa*. But on no account should she have any oil cake while pregnant.

One ounce of salt in the morning and one ounce in the evening should be given to each cow. Clean fresh water must be given three times a day during the cold weather and five times during the hot weather.

Dry cows need protection and shelter from the midday sun, heavy rains, storms and sharp winds, and must be kept in a shed at nights. The sheds and grounds must be kept clean.

When a cow is in calf she must be properly treated.

When a dry cow is brought to the farm, she should be properly bathed with phenyle and water and dried before she is allowed into the farm, and then she must be kept separate from the others for fifteen days.

Each breed of cows should be kept separate, and the bulls kept must be of the same breed as the cows.

Cattle Shows

It was hoped by holding cattle-shows at different centres and giving prizes for the best exhibits people would be encouraged to breed good cattle, but these hopes have not been realized in any great measure.

The following conclusions have been arrived after a detailed study of the subject for many years:

1. It is much better to have several small shows than one big show, for very few people will bring their cows and calves any distance from home. They will bring some good bullocks yoked to carts, on which they and their friends come to the show. They hope to get free fodder and a prize for their bullocks, and in this way pay their expenses to the show.
2. The bullocks and the few cows and calves that are brought to the show are usually purchased from other districts and have not been bred by the owners.

3. Most of the large cattle-shows have degenerated into puppet shows, bioscope and theatrical performances and gambling drives, and very little or no attention is given to the cattle. Most of the money is wasted and very little spent for the benefit of cattle improvement.
4. For the above reasons the object and purpose of cattle-shows are frustrated and money wasted.
5. It would be of more benefit to the people and greater encouragement to cattle-breeding if several local shows were held in villages and stations where people show some interest in the breeding and improvement of their cattle. People from the neighbouring villages, within a radius of three to five miles, may be allowed to bring their cattle to these local shows.
6. These cattle-shows should be held in the early morning or in the evening in convenient places outside of the villages. The judging and prize-giving should be finished in two or three hours and the people allowed to take home their cattle as soon as possible.
7. The people should be instructed in the proper methods of breeding and rearing good cattle, and shown how it would benefit them.
8. Prizes should be given for only the best cows, heifers, bull-calves and young bullocks bred and reared by the owners, or reared from the time they were under a year old to three years old. The prizes should be Rs. 10 and Rs. 8 for the two best milch cows; Rs. 10 and Rs. 8 for the two best heifers, between 2½ and 3 years of age; Rs. 6 and Rs. 5 for the two best female or male calves, under 2 years of age; Rs. 6 and Rs. 5 for the two best young bulls or bullocks, between 2½ and 3 years of age, bred and reared by the owners. The entire cost of such a show will be only Rs. 60, and it is sure such shows would really accomplish the purpose for which they are instituted.

Mr. G.F. Keatinge, Director of Agriculture, Mumbai Presidency, holds the following views on this subject. He says, in his notes on cattle in the Mumbai Presidency,–"It is a debatable question how far cattle-shows stimulate breeding. We have held cattle-shows in connection with cattle fairs and in connection with agricultural shows. At a large cattle fair to which animals are brought for sale, the people can show their cattle in the prize ring without much additional trouble; but they are there mainly to buy and sell, and I do not think that, as a rule, they care much for the show, or that it produces any appreciable result. In the case of a large central show, which is not held in connection with a selling fair, people are sometimes pleased to show their fine bulloks and will come from a long distance to do so; but in many cases the bullocks have been purchased and not bred by the owners, and the giving of prizes can have little effect in stimulating breeding, though it may be a popular adjunct to an agricultural show. Cultivators never, I think, like to bring their cows and young stock from at distance to a show and do so only under compulsion or as a favour. Personally, I think that a show is only useful on a very small scale, in the centre of a good breeding district, and held in connection with some systematic and sustained effort to improve breeding on certain definite lines. Where such an effort is in progress, a series of small shows may well be organized, each confined to a single village. The people will be glad to muster their best cattle outside the village in the early morning, appraise their points, discuss the measures taken for their improvement and receive a few small prizes. The whole, thing is over in a few hours and no trouble has been caused. In the following year the same shows should be held again, and if the people of neighbouring villages show any interest, they may be permitted (but not bothered) to bring their cattle to the show. If after a few years such shows prove a real success, it might be possible to organize a small central show for a limited area (say one Taluk), at which the best cattle at the village shows would be allowed to compete. It is possible that in this way some keenness and competitive spirit might be worked up amongst the breeders, and might lead to more systematic and sustained efforts on their part."

Chapter 32

What Experts Say

Cattle-Breeding in India

Notes taken by Mr. Woodford at a lecture to military farm students delivered by Mr. W. Smith at Ahmedabad

The question of breeding cattle on a scientific basis must in the near future be seriously taken up in India, as the subject is of vital importance to the future of the dairying and agricultural industries.

On approaching this question it will be necessary to divide the problem into three parts:

1. What does India need?
2. What basis have we in India upon which to work?
3. How can we obtain, from the basis available what is needed in India?

What India Needs

The community at large in India needs such a breed of cattle that a large milk yield may be obtained from the female, while the male remains a good draught bullock. The suitability of the male to draught conditions is imperative, since agriculture is the mainstay of India, and in India agriculture depends upon perfect cultivation more than it does in any other country in the world. Other countries have stock-grazing lands, but in this country the grazing areas are comparatively small, invariably neglected, and of poor soil. Gujarat contains the largest milch cattle population per acre in India, and in that district there is no grazing; all fodder is produced by cultivation.

The fact of the necessity of a milking female and a working male from the same breed is obvious, and we are at once confronted by the problem: "Can we produce a breed of cattle which will fulfil these two vital conditions?" Many recognized authorities denied that this was possible, but of those many are coming round to believe that such a combination is possible and that there are no valid reasons against the supposition. In an advanced milking breed, all the maternal instincts and the feeding of young have been developed to the highest pitch, which is an enormous help in breeding a draught bullock, since a first-class milk-giving animal is necessary to rear first-class progeny.

Commercial economy must necessarily be the foundation of the word of breeding. Having attained the type of cattle detailed above there will be two ways of making money open to the farmer and breeder.

(a) By sale of the males or utilizing them on his own lands.

(b) By disposing of the milk from the female.

Hence if a type of animal is produced of which the male realizes in the market a remunerative price, and the female produces a large quantity of milk, the commercial needs of this country will be satisfied.

A dam that is not a good milker cannot produce the above requirements in her sons and daughters. In India, speaking generally, neither the bull nor the cow is looked after. In some districts, the bull is neglected and becomes an incubus on the community, while the cow is cherished for her milk; in other districts the cow runs unwanted and neglected, and the bullock is taken for cultivation. All breeding is just accident and haphazard, and this is the reason that there are 170 million cattle in India where 100 million could do the work, and be sufficient for the needs of the population.

The dual purpose breed for India must mean milk and draught; beef is not wanted as there is no large market for it. The male and female would be each equally useful in their respective lines.

It has been sometimes thought that the most satisfactory way only of the difficulty is to keep the buffalo for milk and the male cow for draught. This means a waste or one sex of each, which is neither businesslike nor economical.

The Basis Upon Which to Work

It may be safely assumed that there is a fairly good plough bullock already, but the female is no milker. The Indian can get almost as good a working bullock as is obtainable in Europe, but cannot get a milker like those of Switzerland and Italy. The Swiss Jura Mountains yellow breed supplies bullocks for the working of the Rhone vineyards at £200 a pair, and show cows of the same breed have given 16,000 lb. of milk per average lactation for three years running. The absence of such conditions as this in India and the want of a good cow account for the presence of the buffalo, but, as before mentioned, the method of keeping buffaloes for milk and bullocks for draught necessitates double the expense and is therefore economically unsound. No country can afford to have its breeding problems based on wrong commercial principles.

The average Indian cow scarcely pays for her feed by her production of milk, so with an animal of this description there is nothing to work upon.

How to Obtain What is Needed

There are only two practicable ways, *viz.*:

(a) To import animals of a good milking strain and introduce that strain into the indigenous cattle.

(b) By the slow process of selection within the country breeds. This will need six generations to obtain appreciable results.

The Importation of Bulls of Milking Strain

This method is quicker and it would seem that the question is solved by a cursory thought. Great care is, however, needed that the draught powers and other characteristics wanted in the half-bred, resulting from the cross between the imported and country strains, may not be destroyed. Certain characteristics, too, which may or may not be known are added from the imported strain, and may not be exactly what are wanted. On the side of the imported strain, which would be bulls of fixed heredity, there is a long line of selection and fixing. On the side of the Indian cow there is no breed, and no fixed characteristics. Hence the sire's qualities predominate and may predominate to an extent almost disastrous, as many of these qualities, such as susceptibility to epidemic diseases, are bad from an Indian point of view.

Take, for example, the high degree of hereditary immunity from the attack of disease of the Indian cow; they have met and struggled with disease so often that resistance has become natural. This immunity is only inherited in two cases out of ten in the half-bred, through the predomination of the fixed line, which carries little or no immunity.

Selection from Indian Cattle

This method would be safe, but it would take 50 years to fix the type, and time cannot be neglected in this case. It has taken the people of Holland 170 years to breed up what is now known as the Holstein Fresian breed of cows. We must be more rapid than this in India. The question is therefore thrown back on imported cattle for the dual purpose. All other countries which have done anything in the line of breeding up cattle have taken breeds from all over the world to get what they wanted; India cannot afford to refuse to do what Japan, Brazil, and Africa have done.

Lines on Which to Work: Mendelian Theory

Breeding in India, with the object of fixing a type of dual purpose cattle for milk and draught, can only be done on the lines of Mendelism, which is, in short, that characteristics are handed on from parents to progeny on an arithmetical basis. Complications arise in this Mendelian ratio, but there is always a rule to cover them.

By working in accordance with the law, it may be possible with scope and care to breed an animal with just those characteristics wanted, and to get rid of those not wanted. To go into particulars, we want the imported line's milking characteristics and the dam's immunity to be dominant.

We also want the spirit of the imported animal and the stamina of the dam's type dominant in the same cross-bred.

The Imported Fixed Line

A criticism of the breeds obtainable for import into India, quickly, decides the question of where the breed that is to bring milk to India may be found. The Jerseys and Guernseys are not suitable, since we already have a good fat percentage in the milk of the indigenous cows. Shorthorn bulls are very costly and the Holstein, with delicate constitution and huge barrel, has no capacity for muscle forming.

Good Ayrshire bulls can be obtained for £40 a head. The breed is the hardiest of all British breeds, their home being in a tough climate. They have the frame from the draught point of view, and the bull is high-spirited. This last quality is of great importance since, when broken to the plough, spirit is needed so that the bullock will pull anything he can move. The Ayrshire seems to fill to the place more completely, especially from the military farms' point of view.

To sum up, we must do away with everything but a type possessing a milking female and a working male, and carrying hereditary immunity and breeding, in accordance with Mendel's theory.

Milch Cattle in India

"The Journal of Dairying"

Where shall we get our milk supply in the future? This important question needs consideration, for it is a well-known fact that milch cattle in India are deteriorating rapidly.

The Government Military Dairies in India are, even now, experiencing a difficulty in obtaining good milch cattle notwithstanding that there are specialists devoting the whole of their time purchasing for this department. They find it almost impossible to get even passable cows, and the position is little better with regard to buffaloes. The difficulty increases each year.

We are well aware that millions of milch cattle exist in India, but what milk do they give? A good average is 5 lb. a day or 750 lb. per lactation, and it is well known that a cow must give 1,250 lb. milk per annum which if sold at two annas per lb. makes it worth while keeping her.

If the *Zamindar* ever makes an investigation into the financial results of keeping cows, probably he will sell out; and with the advance of education, particularly from our Agricultural Colleges in India, these results will soon be known to him.

The causes of the deterioration of the cattle in India is that thousands of the best cows are ruined by the milkmen in the cities and sold to butchers. If the milkmen in Indian cities could be prevented from ruining good milch cows and killing their calves, something could be done to improve the cattle. In *Dairying and Dairy Farming,* under his article entitled "The Indian Cow as a Dairy

Animal," Mr. Reeves shows very clearly what casual, methods of breeding cattle prevail here. He says:

"The common system of breeding (if it can be called, a system) prevailing in this country is to allow a number of bulls, in each city or village, to roam about and serve *ad. lib.* These bulls are owned by no particular individual but by the community at large, each and every one assisting in feeding them; and it is a common and everyday sight in the bazaars of Indian cities to see these bulls going from house to house and shop to shop to receive their daily allowance of food from the owners. Owing to their non-fastidious taste (eating any thing offered to them) they are always in good condition."

"They usually feed in the early morning, and about 9 A.M. the cows of each and every owner are turned out into the streets (often from the house in which the owner himself lives), where the bulls join them, and the whole saunter off to graze somewhere outside the city, or, if grazing is not available, to some shady spot where they remain until evening, when the cows return to their homes, the bulls remaining outside in the bazaars generally. The city or village herds are very mixed and poorly developed, owing to this indiscriminate breeding; in some few districts, however, there are particular types, and this has given us the few breeds we have, which, although not pure, are distinct from the mongrel-bred cattle of many parts of the country."

"The religious belief of the native allows of breeding from maimed and useless animals, whose progeny swells the enormous number of wretchedly developed animals in the country who only breed and spread disease. The Hindoo does all in his power to prevent cows from being slaughtered, and in every large city there are one or more depositories kept up by private subscription where maimed and old cattle are placed to escape the butcher and so finish their days in the natural way."

"Only a few days ago the writer visited one of these places in a small city in Scinde where 950 head of such cattle are kept at an expense of about £6,000 a year. However much more beneficial would it be to the community if this amount was devoted to improving the breed of their cattle?"

India cannot possibly stand this strain even with organized breeding. From the above remarks it is evident that the milking strains of cattle must go on deteriorating until the milking qualities are almost extinct, and in fact cows will scarcely be able to bring up calves even for draught purposes.

Cannot something be done to stem this tide of destruction of an animal that is so necessary to the welfare of the country?

The question is, who is to investigate this matter? Will not our Indian friends cooperate and form societies for the prevention of this wholesale destruction of *good cattle* in our cities, by purchasing up all the best dry cows of milking breeds and sending them to some places where they could be kept with good bulls and they and their progeny well tended, and thus save the situation indicated? They could also form areas in districts for breeding up the milking qualities by the same process. If the milking qualities of cattle deteriorate, so will cattle for draught purposes. Many of our chief administrators are well versed in the best methods of breeding in England, and if they will turn their expert knowledge and administrative ability to this subject they would confer a boon on the country that every Indian gentleman would appreciate. The difficulty is to form an ideal method of carrrying out a scheme for this revolution, but the master-minds of our Governors, assisted by their professional experts, could perhaps evolve a scheme that would at least make a beginning.

The Government Military Dairies are arranging for themselves, and should, with the policy now being pursued, become self-supporting in a year or two, particularly if the young stock are immunized from rinderpest. Their methods are, however, unsuitable for the country generally, but would help considerably as a guide in formulating a scheme for cooperative societies when. organized.

The worst part of the situation at present is that the people always look to Government to carry out improvements, and one fears there is little chance of any improvement unless Local Governments do undertake to make a start. The Imperial Government has made a move in the right direction by establishing the Dairy Institute at Bangalore where substantial works are being done with regard to Dairy Farming, Animal Husbandry and Breeding. The Local Governments should make several small experimental cattle breeding Farms and Dairies in different Districts on the line of Dacca and Rungpore in Bengal. If considerable progresses are made by these farms on the practical side, then Indian gentlemen will come forward with financial assistance, in fact it can be asserted that there would be no difficulty in this respect. The eagerness of the Local Governments is manifested by their creation and appointment, in most of the Provinces, of Live Stock Experts: who will work up the details of cattle-breeding and improvement and the people, who are very much conservative in their ideas, will greatly benefit by such expert advices.

Breeding Milch Catttle

By Captain G.H. Frost

In the discussion on Mendel's law it was also indicated that the best way to secure a given type, so that it would be transmitted with reasonable certainty from parent to offspring, was to select for mating those animals possessing in the most perfect form the characters which we wish to secure in the offspring. Selection is, therefore, the all-powerful agent in controlling the characters of farm animals generally.

Inferior animals should be eliminated from breeding, as they tend to reproduce themselves. On the other hand, superior offspring should be selected for breeding, as they also tend to reproduce themselves, and to show still further improvement. Thus, one of the primary objects of selection is to improve the ancestry, preventing, so far as possible, the birth of unwelcome individuals not suited to the purposes of man. The animal breeder can prevent the birth of unprofitable individuals approximately in proportion as he is skilled in selection.

This affords the breeder an opportunity to influence the character and type of his animals, as only superior ones should be retained for breeding purposes. While selection is a very important factor in establishing type, it does not greatly reduce variability. This necessitates watchfulness on the part of the breeder, and he must eliminate all animals from breeding that do not meet the requirements of the given type.

Standards of Excellence in Selection

The breeder must have a definite ideal or a standard of excellence for his guidance in selecting his breeding animals. Among the great run of variation which every breeder will encounter, he must know which are useful, which are fanciful, and which are mere novelties. The standard must not be altered by fancy considerations or by novelties, no matter how curious or attractive.

The standard must be fixed in advance. It should be wisely chosen in the light of what is needed. Due consideration should be given to every influence. Once chosen, however, the standard should be preserved unchanged. Blood lines must be kept pure, not only within the breed, but within the strain or family with which we are working. This is emphasized by the law of ancestral heredity, and by the fact that, no matter what the parent, the offspring tends strongly towards the average of the race to which it belongs.

On the other hand, the sire has a decided advantage over the dam in that he can influence large numbers in a breeding season, whereas the dam can control but one, or at most a few as is the case of swine.

Influence of the Sire

From the foregoing it is evident that the upper limit of the sire is comparatively very high and the dam very low. The statement is often made that the sire is half the herd, whereas he is far more than that. He is one-half the herd the first generation, three-quarters the second, seven-eighths the third, and fifteen-sixteenths the fourth. So powerful is the influence of the sire that if careful selection be maintained for a few generations, he will mould the character of the entire herd. This fact should warn us of the necessity of exercising extreme care in the selection of the sire.

While the influence of climate and locality is great and the factors at work are exceedingly complex, yet from a practical point of view we may consider the food supply and more favourable conditions generally, such as sufficient shelter; proper care, including training and developing, as the more important causes of variation.

Care and Management

In the breeding of animals the conditions of environment are changed or enlarged by man, who provides his animals with favourable conditions. The improvement derived from proper care and management is not fully appreciated by the average breeder.

Food Supply

The food supply is of prime importance in effecting improvement among animals. No other conditions influence development to a greater extent. Large breeds are developed from small ones largely by increasing the food supply. In addition to the increase in size, there is also an increase in the constitutional vigour when the animal is well fed.

In order to secure increased development of all of the productive functions the animal must be supplied with more food than is required for the performance of the normal functions.

Chief among these are suitable food; protection from cold, heat, enemies and all annoying influences; proper management and suitable preparation, including training and developing.

The intending breeder should make a careful study of the situation, taking account of the market demands, the general environment as well as his own limitations, and select the breed best suited to his particular conditions, as certain breeds are not well adapted to certain conditions. A good example of the principle involved is observed in the case of dairy cattle. A careful study of the dairy industry reveals the fact that in general large cows are replacing small ones in localities where the land is level and easily grazed; while small cows are replacing large ones in hilly districts where grazing is difficult.

In selecting animals for breeding, constitutional vigour is one of the most important characteristics to be considered. No animal lacking in thrift should find its way into the breeding herd, no matter how excellent, no matter what the pedigree, and no matter how high may be the record of performance.

While little understood, enough is known regarding prepotency to enable the skilled breeder to select animals possessing it with a reasonable degree of certainty. This is specially true when records of performance are available.

Prepotency is considered from two points of view: first, breed prepotency, by which is meant that animals of a breed are all possessed of much power in transmitting the characters of the breed; and, secondly, individual prepotency, in which the individual has much power in transmitting its characters to the offspring.

In fact, the prepotency of the pure-bred over the common animal is the significant factor in breed prepotency, as it enables us to transform quickly the common animal to the type of the breed from which pure-bred males have been selected. In this connection it must be remembered that some breeds are much more prepotent than others, and hence will effect changes more rapidly.

Thus the breeder who wishes to give his animals the most benefit possible of good blood at the least expense will, of course, provide it through the sires' side. For purely economic reasons, therefore, sires in general are prepotent over dams.

Improvement of Slow Process

While remarkable advance has been gained in increasing the efficiency of such class of farm animals, yet the improvement of economic characters is a slow process, requiring years of careful study and patient effort. When selection and improvement are limited to a single character, advancement may be fairly rapid at first, but as maximum efficiency is approached, the rate of increase rapidly diminishes, and improvement calls for greater effort on the part of the breeder.

Methods Employed

From the foregoing discussions on improvement due to selection based on records of performance, improvement due to selection, the result of prepotency, as well as improvement due to accumulative development, it must be clear, that efficiency depends largely on selection; that judicious selection depends on an exact knowledge of development or performance, and that the degree of development depends on the environment, including training, management and the like.

Since the system to be employed will depend largely upon the purpose, the breeder should first of all have a clear idea of just what he is trying to do, and an accurate knowledge of the limitations of the various systems, so that he may employ the proper one to achieve his purpose.

An attempt to improve those for immediate use may be defined as *herd improvement*; while the improvement of those for breeding purposes may be defined as *breed improvement*.

In herd improvement the object is the betterment of the individual. This is purely commercial. It is, perhaps, the cheapest and most convenient of all forms of breeding and productive of the most rapid gains. On the other hand, in breed improvement the object is the betterment of the entire strain or race.. This is creative and constructive. It is, perhaps, the most expensive, although of the very highest style of finished breeding and calls for intelligent, painstaking effort, as in this case the breeder is a true leader in the improvement of types and breeds of farm animals.

This constitutes animal improvement in the true sense of the term and is the highest system of finished breeding. It has the disadvantage in that it is rather, costly, especially when the purpose is to produce something better than ever existed before. This is because so few individuals materially excel their predecessors on their contemporaries, and so few of these can be relied upon to propagate their own excellence.

Grading

This consists in mating a common animal with a purely bred one. The pure-bred may be either sire or dam; but for economic reasons it is usually the sire.

There is no cheaper, quicker or more thorough way to become familiar with a breed than through a familiarity with its grades. Further, in a few generations grades may be so improved as to be practically equal to pure-breds for immediate consumption, although they will be worthless, for breeding purposes.

Cross-Breeding

This system rendered a valuable service in forming new breeds. Indeed, but few breeds of farm animals have been evolved without more or less cross-breeding among the foundation animals.

Developing the Heifer

The young heifer that is to remain in the dairy herd should be given extra care from birth, in order that she may be well grown by the time she is sexually mature. To develop a high-producing cow it is important that she be bred at an early age and this can be done to advantage only in case she is well grown. The claim is made by some persons that the demands made on the young heifer by the growing foetus, together with her own growth, are too severe, and that she is likely to he stunted. On the other hand, experience indicates that the constant recurring periods of restrum check growth, and that the condition of pregnancy has a stimulating effect. The assimilation seems to be improved, and if the heifer be supplied with an abundance of nutritious food she will make a greater growth during pregnancy than otherwise.

The breeding (serving) of the well grown heifer at 21 months of age has much to commend it. In the first place, unbred heifers are in oestrum two or three days every three weeks, and it is at such times that reproductive organs are likely to become infected with the germ of contagious abortion, which may cause sterility, or in case the heifer conceives, it may produce abortion. Thus the animal bred early in life is likely to escape this infection and prove a regular breeder. In the second place, it is possible to develop the milk-secreting organs of a heifer much more perfectly than of an older animal.

The secreting of milk is a kind of habit, and the earlier in life the young heifer becomes accustomed to it the better producer she will make. Once giving milk, she should be kept at it as long as possible. The cow that dries off after secreting milk a few months is unprofitable. The heifer should not be bred a second time until rather late, as the effect, of again becoming pregnant has a tendency to decrease the flow of milk. During the first lactation the object is to keep her in milk as long as possible, in order to develop a persistent milker, rather than to encourage a high production for a short time and then dry her off, as is the usual practice.

Therefore, to secure maximum development in farm animals, both young and old, the management must be as favourable as possible to advance all of the potentialities of the individual.

The efficiency of the individuals in hand depends upon vigorous selection, based on maximum development of all the potentialities with which the individual has been endowed. Further selection under such conditions purifies the strain, family, or breed by the elimination of all individuals not possessing the desirable characters.

For, in the main, the environment controls the development and directs selection, and selection governs individual efficiency and purifies the strains, families, and breeds of our farm animals.

Rearing of Calves in India

By W. Reeves

Possibly too much cannot be written on this subject at this period. Owing to the impotation of British and Australian pure bred stock, and the high prices and increasing difficulty of purchasing good cattle, calves on our farms are much more valuable than heretofore–in fact, at one time it was very doubtful whether they were worth rearing; there is little doubt now.

If the conditions of this country. were the same as those of Europe, Australia and America, this article would no doubt be superfluous, for volumes have been written on the subject, both scientifically and as the result of generations of experience, but these only apply to those countries and their stock. In India we have not the same conditions nor have we the physically hard-bred stock such as are found in temperate climates. We have also the buffalo calf to rear, about which little or nothing has yet been written. The information given is chiefly confined to the rearing of weaned buffalo and cow calves.

The calf should be taken away at birth (This can be done in India only with a cow with her first calf.-I.T.), care being taken that the mother does not see it, so that she may not worry or go in search of it afterwards, which is likely to upset cow and calf. She ought to be blindfolded, the calf when taken away should be carefully wiped with pieces of soft dry cloth and then sponged over with warm water, until clean, and then dried by light brisk rubbing with sponge clothes kept for the purpose.

Wash out the mouth with clean water and bind up the navel cord tightly with carbolized silk thread, after washing in an antiseptic solution.

When properly cleaned, place it in a dry spot free from cold draughts or excessive heat, and away from other calves.

Put a little bedding under it, taking care that it is free from insect life, for, if it is not, your troubles will commence right away, for calves can never thrive if worried with parasites.

Do not be in a hurry to give it its first feed, allow it to become strong on its legs and gain a good appetite before introducing its initial repast, which should consist of two or three pounds (according to size of calf) of colostrum straight from the mother. It now has to be taught to feed by the aid of the fingers–this is done by taking a little milk in the palm of the hand, inserting one or two fingers into its mouth and allowing the milk to run down them; in a short time it will commence to suck, when the vessel should be raised and the hand lowered into the milk, and the calf induced to suck the milk up the fingers. Be careful not to press on its nose with the hand, or allow it to suck the fingers when not in the milk, or it will suck in air and probably bring on indigestion and scours.

The same should be given three times per day for a week, at 6 A.M., 1 P.M., and 8 P.M. Take care that it does not lose flesh at this period, or it will be found difficult to regain. it. (Such young calves should be given smaller quantities at a time and fed five times a day until four weeks old.–S.N.S.).

It should now be moved to a class of calves from one week to a month old, these being quite apart from those of other ages, and where many are kept, the cow-calves should be separate from the buffalo-calves.

Meals will now consist of 1½ lb. pure and 1½ lb. separated milk (Horlick's malted milk-which is very light, good and equally efficacious.–S.N.S.), with the addition of a little scalded barley meal, boiled linseed, and *gurh*, at 6 A.M. and 8 P.M., 2 lb. of separated and a little of the admixture at 1 P.M. (Give smaller quantities five times a day.–S.N.S.)

The feed should be prepared for this class in bulk by scalding the barley meal with separated milk heated to pasteurizing temperature, adding the linseed which has been boiled overnight, and, mixing in the *gurh* and pure milk, stir the whole well and allow it to cool to about 90°. ½ barley (or gram) meal, 2 oz. linseed, 2 oz. *gurh*, per calf per diem will be sufficient for this class. Always keep in mind that buffalo-calves require at least two pounds per day more than cow-calves, so the feed should be divided out accordingly.

It will be found that this diet keeps the bowels free, and there is little chance of the milk clogging and curdling in the stomach as is the case when pure milk is fed alone. While in this class, the calf should be taught to feed without the aid of the fingers; this is done by occasionally drawing away the fingers from its mouth until it realizes that they are no longer a necessity. Tie up each calf for half an hour after feeding to prevent them sucking at each other. When a month old it should be again moved, this time to a class whose ages range from one to three months, and its ration is again changed to 4 lb. separated milk with the addition of barley (or gram) meal, linseed, and *gurh*, as before at 6 A.M. and 8 P.M., and 2 lb. separated milk and a little of the admixture at 1 P.M. (Feed four times a day and give smaller quantities–I.T.). The feed should be prepared as for the former class. Individual feeding should be no longer necessary now, the feed should fed in troughs that can easily be cleaned, preferably of glazed earthenware, or galvanized iron, and they should be carefully cleaned after each meal. This also applies to all other vessels used for feeding. At this period the calf will commence to forage for itself, and to aid it in this, an extra half pound of barley meal or a little bran, mixed with sweet-chaffed hay, should be given, and also a little green fodder if it is available.

At the age of three months the milk diet may be dispensed with, and it should now be moved to a class between three and six months old, and to obviate falling off in condition after taking it off milk diet butter-milk and any waste separated milk should be fed to this class. (At this age the calf should be fed three times a day-early in the morning, at 1 P.M., and again at 7 or 8 P.M.).

"Do not spoil your ship for a halfpenny worth of paint" at this period and think your calf can now thrive on a bit of withered grass or coarse fodder. It requires more nourishment now than before, only in a different form. Feed it well and you will have it in your milking herd earning its feed while the badly fed ones are still calves. One hears it said that "it does not pay to feed calves and young stock well in this country." It certainly never pays to feed them badly. What sort of a cow can you expect from a badly fed calf? Certainly not one that will do you any credit. If you have selected those for keeping from good stock it will pay you over and over again to treat them well. The point of greatest importance in the rearing of calves is the housing of them, all your feed, care, and attention will be mitigated if your housing is bad and does not allow of good sanitary measures being carried out.

Nearly all the diseases that calves are susceptible to are introduced through the medium of insanitary sheds. A shed for the plains needs to be open on at least two sides to admit of fresh air passing through both day and night. If it becomes necessary in the cold weather to close it up at night, this may be done by hanging tarpaulins as curtains, so that it can be easily opened up again in the day to allow of it being well aired.

It should have a good floor impervious to moisture, brick on edge grouted with thin cement being the best, unless good flagstones are cheaper, and it should be regrouted when it shows any interstices. Calves can never be successfully reared on *kutcha* floors, and where these are a necessity in the case of runs, the runs should be changed occasionally and the floors dug out to the depth of a foot and new earth or sand put in.

Floors should be washed down morning and evening, the calves being turned out while this is being done. The most common diseases amongst calves in this country are scours, hoose, ringworm and mange, but these need not be feared if proper attention is given to good housing careful feeding, cleanliness, and prevention of exposure to extremes of heat or cold.

Remember that a rupee spent in prevention will go as far as twenty spent on cures, with calves.

Personal-attention to ensure the above being *regularly* attended to is of great importance. The above measures or any other good system is nullified by irregularity and unequal amounts of milk.

Plenty of water, exercise and lumps of rock salt to lick are very necessary.

Calf-raising is a necessity on every dairy farm. It is the only economical and safe method of keeping a herd. Culling the herd is the surest system of upbuilding.

The Royal Agricultural Society of England has been conducting some experiments on the rearing of calves, and has issued a report of the results. These experiments were carried out with several batches of animals, divided into five groups, and over a period of nine weeks. The different kinds of food were as follow:

Cod-liver oil and separated milk; calf meal, gruel containing linseed; oatmeal and separated milk; whole crushed oats with separated milk. The whole result of the experiments may be summed up in one statement that the crushed oats and separated milk gave the best returns. This is very instructive indeed, and is all in favour of the use of home-grown food, as both the oats and separated milk may be produced on the farm. The present writer has just been informed by one of his neighbours that the best food he has discovered for the growth of calves after the first month of milk-feeding is over, is a mixture of oats and beans. The beans are only partly chewed and regurgitated and chewed over again in the ordinary way that the cud is treated, and thus the function of rumination is carried on with this particular kind of food.

In these trials of the "Royal" it was found chat not only did the crushed oats and separated milk have the best effect on the young animals up to weaning time, but the animals throve better afterwards when turned out, to grass than those of any other group. It is pointed out by Dr. Voelker, who issued the report, that a good start to the young animals seems to enable them to carry on right ahead after a particular treatment is dropped, and it is intended to carry on these experiments with these same animals till they are fatted for the butcher, and to keep a record of their growth and development as against the food during the time.

A Useful Calf Meal

If, however, any one still prefers to use a calf meal, that is, one that must be made up with warm water and fed as a gruel or thin soup as milk substitute, then the following recipe will be found to be an exceedingly useful one for home-made purposes: 7 lb. oatmeal; 7 lb. linseed meal; 7 lb. locust bean meal; 2 lb. arrowroot. The arrowroot (cheap commercial form) is for the purpose of preventing scouring; and the writer had the recipe from one of the most successful calf rearers he ever had the privilege of meeting. [Gram or wheat meal (slightly parched) will do very well instead of locust bean meal–S.N.S.].

Rearing of Calves of Government Military Farms

"The Journal of Dairying"

1. In the past it has been the custom at most military dairy farms to rear all heiger calves from both cows and buffaloes with a view to their being added to the milking herd, but the greatly increased prices of feeding stuffs in the past few years call for a revision of this policy, as the yield record of many farm-reared animals has proved that they do not repay the cost of rearing. In future, therefore, managers will only rear country-bred heifer calves from cows showing an average yield of 2,500 lb. per annum of over, and buffalow heifer calves from animals yielding 3,000 lb. per year or over. All half-bred-English and Indian-heifer calves will be reared as formerly.

2. As regards bull calves for stud purposes at all dairies where imported bulls are not used four cow bulls will be reared annually for every 100 milch cows kept oil the farm. These will be selected from the best milking animals in the herd which drop male calves, and no such bulls to be reared unless the dam has an average record of 3,000 lb. or over per annum.

   Buffalo stud bulls to the extent of 2 per cent of the milking herd and from dams yielding 4,000 lb. per year or over will be reared at all farms.

3. In the past managers have often been deterred from feeding sucking calves generously owing to the fact that on reaching maturity so many proved to be poor milkers, but if good bulls are used it may safely be assumed that the progeny of animals giving the above specified yields will repay the cost of proper rearing from birth, and in future managers of all dairies will be held responsible that the calves and young stock being reared either as stud bulls or for the milking herd are kept in first-class condition at all times, and that they are matured as early as possible.

4. All calves to be reared for stud or milking purposes must be set apart at birth and kept separate throughout their existence from those to be sold or reared for bullocks. Past experience has proved that we cannot afford under present conditions to prevent the *gowallas* from having the calf beside the country-bred cow at milking time, but it should be the aim of the management to permit the calf to draw as little milk as possible from its dam, so that in fixing rations for sucking calves no account whatever need be taken of anything but the rations fed from the pail.

5. Not only is it essential that all calves to be reared should be kept apart from the rest of the herd, but it is also necessary that these animals should be housed, and fed in pens according to their age. Thus animals. under one month should be together, animals from one to three months should form another lot, from three to six months a third pen, and those from six to nine months should be housed together; after nine months they should be classed as young stock.

6. In fixing rations for young calves for rearing it must be recognized that nothing can entirely take the place of new milk for the first month, and for the first week of its, existence every calf set apart for rearing shall receive not less than 6 lb. of new milk per *diem*. During this period nothing but the new milk will be given. For the next three weeks, a mixture of not less than 2 lb. new milk and 4 lb. separated milk will be fed with the addition of a small quantity of finely ground barley meal, or maize meal or linseed cake meal. About six ounces daily of any of these meals or a mixture of them should be added to the milk and the whole boiled together and fed in the form of gruel flavoured with either *gurh* or salt.

   From the age of one month no new milk need be given, but if separated milk is available it may be fed boiled with a mixture of the above meals in the form of porridge or gruel to the extent of 8 lb. of separated milk and 1½ lb. of meal per day from 1 to 3 months, and 10 lb. milk and 3 lb. meal per day from 3 to 6 months. The solid part of these rations should of course, be gradually increased, as for instance ¾ lb. meal would be sufficient for a calf one month old, but 2 lb. could with safety be fed at 3 months old. The full quantities of separated milk should be fed throughout the periods mentioned, but the quantities of meal given are average figures. From 6 to 9 months, the meal rati on should be increased to 4 lb. fed in the same manner with 10 lb. separated milk in the form of gruel.

   Where separated milk is not available, the quantities of meal to be given must be increased by 1 lb. for every 10 lb. separated milk stipulated, and the meal must be made into a fine gruel by boiling with water to which 1 oz. *gurh* per animal per day is added, when separated milk is not available maize meal may not be fed.

   All calves up to 9 months old should be fed three times a day, and in addition to the above rations they should get as much green and dry fodder as they will eat. It is absolutely necessary that all reared calves should be taught to drink from the pail at birth, and it is not sufficient that managers give an order that these animals are to be fed in such and such a manner or on such and such a ration. They must personally see that the correct rations are issued, that they are properly cooked and prepared, and that the animals actually partake of them.

7. Separated milk in the form of gruel must in all cases be fed fresh and sweet. Sour or curdled milk must not be fed to young calves. Meals used for gruel must be fresh and wholesome and the feeding troughs should be thoroughly cleaned out before the next feed is given. Stale gruel may be fed to adult stock. Vessels in which gruel is made and served including feeding troughs must be kept scrupulously clean.
8. In addition to proper feeding of young calves, it is of great importance that they should get proper exercise and that they should be cleanly and comfortably housed. The walls of all calf-sheds and railings of all calf-pens should be lime-washed once a week and lime, freely sprinkled over the floors at the same time. By proper feeding, scrupulous cleanliness, and frequent lime-washing only we can keep tour herds free of the skin diseases which are so prevalent in this country.
9. Calves which have been selected for rearing owing to the milk yield of their dams but which themselves show unmistakable signs of "bad doers," and which do not thrive, should be transferred to ordinary stock on the orders of the Assistant Directors, to whose notice cases of this sort should be brought at their inspections.
10. Calves not up to the standard for rearing as stud bulls or milkers should be sold as soon as weaned and they must in all cases be kept strictly separate from the "reared animals." They should not even be allowed to graze together. It should be clearly understood that the rations set forth in this letter apply solely to calves being reared to join the farm herd.

Artificial Milk of Calves and Pigs

(Terrion *Acad. des Science*), November 18th, 1930, gives the following formula for making an artificial milk which satisfies the protein mineral and vitamin requirements of normal milk and less inclined to cause digestive troubles in calves:

Tapioca meal 112 grams (a gram = about 17 grains); pea meal 75 grams; extract of malt 13 grams; calcium citrate 2 grams; sodium chloride 1 gram; sodium bicarbonate 6.25 grams, and water 1 litre (litre = about 1¾ pint).

For pigs no ill effects arise from the use of this mixture alone. In calves it is used with equal parts of raw milk.

Improvement of Cattle in Bengal

By E. Shearer, M.A., B.Sc.

From the point of view of climate and of agriculture, Bengal may be said to be divided into three main tracts: (1) Lower Bengal, (2) Bihar, and (3) Chota Nagpur and the hilly portions of Orissa. The conditions in the latter tract are in every way widely divergent from those in the rest of the province, and in this article only Lower Bengal and Bihar will come under review. Speaking generally, in both these regions the soil is extremely, fertile and the rainfall is usually plentiful or sufficient. The cultivation is consequently of an intensive character. In Lower Bengal, where the rainfall is heavy and well distributed over the year, wet crops, such as paddy and jute, are principally grown. In Bihar, with a lighter rainfall, paddy is usually confined except where there is canal irrigation, as in Shahabad, to the lower-lying lands, but a great variety of dry crops is grown, much of the land ordinarily bearing both a *kharif* and a *rabi* crop in the same year. The population which is almost wholly agricultural is very dense, often exceeding 1,000 to the square mile.

In this country the common experience is that the quality of the cattle varies inversely with the intensiveness of the cultivation, and hence it is hardly surprising that Bengal cattle are the worst in India. It is almost entirely a question of food supply. For many generations the cattle have been consistently starved, and the result is seen in the degenerate specimens existing today. Over the greater portion of the Bengal plains, grazing is very limited. In the Shahabad, North Darbhanga and North Champaran districts of Bihar there are still considerable expanses of waste land, and there some quite good cattle and certainly the best in Bihar are to be found. With the pressure of population these grazing areas are continually being encroached on. In Darbhanga district they are said to have contracted twenty-five per cent. within the last few years, and in Shababad the opening of the Sone Canal has brought a great deal of what was previously waste land under cultivation. In most of Bihar, and still more in Lower Bengal, grazing supplies only an infinitesimal portion of the food required by the enormous numbers of cattle. The remainder is very inadequately supplied from the fodder available from the field crops. In Bihar the average cultivator's bullock is a starved, stunted, weedy-looking beast. It is active but quite incapable of hard or prolonged work.

The tillage implements are of the lightest character and only the easy working nature of the soil makes decent cultivation at all possible. Even as it is, by better tillage alone, Bihar could probably be made to yield fifty per cent better crops. The cows are worse comparatively than the bullocks, for the latter have the first call on the food supply. They usually yield a negligible quantity of milk; and the young stock, especially the young female stock, are consequently starved from the beginning. In Lower Bengal we find the same state of things, only in a more intensified degree. The cattle are probably of the same stock originally as those in Bihar, but they have become still more diminutive and tillage implements have been reduced in size correspondingly.

If, then, we except Shahabad and certain portions of North Bihar, where a fair number of moderately good cattle is produced, the condition of the cattle in Bengal could not well be worse. The Government has recognized the necessity of doing something to remedy this state of affairs, and within the last few years herds of selected cows have been established at Siripur, and, by arrangement with the Government of India, at Pusa. for the purpose of breeding bulls of a superior type for distribution in the province. The cows for these herds have been selected by the Civil Veterinary Department from the Shahabad district chiefly. The object is to produce compact, well-built bulls with good bone, but not too large since they, will have to mate with small cows. The cows have not been selected for their milking powers. The sole object at present is to produce bulls which will beget better work cattle.

It may be asked how far the method adopted for the improvement of cattle in Bengal is likely to succeed. There is no doubt that there is a great scarcity of good bulls all over the province, and all that Pusa and Siripur can supply will be eagerly sought for. Such bulls also should have a considerable effect in raising the standard of work cattle in the districts which they serve, for the cultivator usually does the best he can by his male young stock. On the other hand, the area of the province, is enormous, and at the best only a comparatively small portion of it can ever be supplied with these better bred bulls. Unless the cultivators can learn the lesson of what can be done by selection and breeding, and themselves carry on the work, little permanent improvement can be looked for. The weakness of the present method of improvement (apart from the impossibility of supplying more than a fraction of the number of bulls required) is that all the attention is being concentrated on the bulls, while no account is being taken of the cows. However good the bulls may be, no good stock can be produced if the cows continue to be starved and neglected as they are now; and there is little doubt that they will continue to be starved and neglected until the cultivator obtains a better cow. The fact is that at present the average cow is in such a wretched states that the cultivator cannot afford to feed her better than he does. Practically, the only return which she gives for her feed is her calf, and that is not enough. What he wants is a good milch cow which will not only rear a calf but leave a substantial surplus of milk to her owner. Such a cow he is prepared to pay for and prepared to feed. It is surprising how little more a good milch cow eats than a bad one. She is simply a more efficient animal.

To produce for Bengal a type of cow which will be a good milker, and at the same time breed work cattle of the type required for the province, does not seem to be impossible of realization. It may take many years, but until such a type is produced, strongly believe that on substantial or permanent improvement in the cattle will be effected.

Part 2

Chapter 1

Diseases of Cattle, Goats and Sheep

There are many diseases of a very serious type that cattle are subjected to. Some of them are very contagious and most fatal.

These diseases are commonly met with in India, and unless proper preventive and curative measures are promptly adopted on the appearance of any contagious disease in the district, or in the herd, one must not be surprised if most of his cattle are attacked and destroyed by it.

Cattle when properly cared for and fed seldom become ill.

When they are over-fed or badly fed, they become unhealthy and suffer much from disease.

Some of the diseases are contracted from contagion, while others are solely attributable to mismanagement in the care and feeding.

The causes of the different diseases are herein fully explained; and in most cases the causes can be prevented by ordinary care and watchfulness, so cattle owners in most cases will have only themselves to blame if any of these diseases attack their stock.

Hay, straw, *bhoosa*, bran, etc., must be stored for seasons of drought, inundation, heavy rains, or where cattle-plague may be prevailing. Generally, cattle are let loose to pick up what they can as food; and very often they eat acrid or poisonous plants and grass. In India, after the inundation subsides, the submerged pastures are very injurious and cause disease.

If cattle are sent out to graze during the rains, great care must be taken that the lands are properly drained.

Cattle cannot remain healthy if exposed to heavy rains or kept on inundated lands, or are not sheltered from the heat of the midday sun and cold damp winds at night.

Disease is very often caused from the foul water the cattle are allowed to drink.

Rinderpest is the most contagious disease among cattle in India, and is very fatal. From 30 to 50 per cent of the cattle attacked die.

Black-quarter, Anthrax, and Haemorrhagic Septicaemia in cattle, and Braxy in sheep, are undoubtedly contagious in India, and very fatal; an animal seldom recovers. Braxy in sheep is, however, rarely met with in India.

The following rules should be strictly adhered to:

1. When cattle, sheep, or goats are purchased at a fair, they should be always treated as having been exposed to contagion, as cattle and sheep are brought to the fair from all directions, and in one direction or other rinderpest or foot-and-mouth disease or other diseases, very probably, have lately been or are prevailing.
2. When cattle, sheep, or goats are being moved from one locality to another they should not be allowed to mix with others en route, and should never be kept at night in or near any *serai* or bazaar, as a *serai* is often contaminated by being occupied, or having lately been occupied by diseased animals; they should travel in the cool time of the day-this should be particularly observed during the hot weather; and they ought not to travel more than eight or ten miles during the twenty-four hours. They should be frequently watered and well fed.
3. When cattle, sheep, or goats are purchased at a fair or elsewhere, they should, on being brought to the purchaser's premises, be kept by themselves, and not allowed to mix with the old cattle of the farm at pasture or watering time, or at any time. They should be kept by themselves for at least one to two weeks in order to have proof whether they are affected with disease or not.

During that time the newly purchased animals should be carefully inspected morning and evening, and if any contagion appears among them, the affected animals should be at once isolated, and the remainder separated into small lots and picketed at some distance apart. At the end of the above period if no disease has appeared among them they may be safely pastured and kept with the other cattle.

4. When cattle are travelling, or are moved from one district to another, they are exposed to contagion and are liable to contract disease; therefore, on their arrival at home they should be carefully examined, and if they have passed through an infected district, they should be kept separated for some time.
5. When disease, supposed to be of a contagious nature, appears among cattle, sheep, or goats, the first important duty is to separate the sick from the healthy animals.
6. Carefully examine all the animals, and remove to the hospital any showing the slightest symptoms of disease.
7. During the prevalence of contagion, divide the healthy cattle into several lots, making each lot as small in number as space will permit. Picket the cattle in such lots a good distance apart, and to windward of the sick cattle. Frequently examine each lot, and remove at once any animal in the least unwell. By steadily a adopting this plan, the disease will be found in few days to exist only among one or two lots, and by at once removing to the hospital any becoming sick, the disease will speedily be arrested in spreading through the herd. Each lot should be kept isolated from other cattle for about two or three weeks after being put by themselves, or after the last animal of the lot affected has been removed.
8. The hospital should be at a good distance from the cow-shed, enclosed by a strong fence. The attendants and the sick cattle must not be permitted to leave the enclosure. Food and water may be taken to the attendants and cattle, but no forage or water, litter, or clothing, or anything should be taken from the hospital. Dogs should not be allowed to go to and from the hospital as they will carry contagion.

9. The dry litter, etc., of the hospital should be burnt inside the hospital area, and the moist dung and discharges, etc., should be frequently removed from the stalls and buried in pits dug in the hospital premises far away from the stall. These pits should be six feet or more deep, and should be filled with the wet litter, dung, etc., of the hospital up to within two feet of the surrounding ground surface, and then quicklime and good fresh earth should be used to fill up the remaining two feet.
10. The stalls, walls, etc., and ground of the hospital should be scrupulously cleaned by frequent sweeping and washing, and after every cleansing, some disinfecting powder, or phenyle, lime, wood ashes, or even dry earth, should be plentifully scattered over the floors and ground, and the woodwork and walls should be first washed and then white-washed with lime.
11. The hospital should be well ventilated. Sulphur fumigation should be daily carried out for an hour or so in the hospital building; and at this time the doors and windows should be closed, and the ventilators only kept partly open.
12. The sick cattle should be kept scrupulously clean and have thin rice, wheat, linseed and sattoo-gruel, and fresh green grass as diet. The healthy cattle should also be kept on soft and laxative food, as cattle fed on hard, dry food have the disease in a more severe form than those fed on laxative fodder.
13. When these contagious diseases have prevailed among cattle or sheep, they should not be allowed to pasture or be kept with unaffected herds until one or two weeks have expired after the last case of disease occurring among the affected lot.
14. Animals that recover should be well washed with warm water and soap prior to being removed from the hospital. Phenyle should be added to the warm water in the proportion of one wineglassful to a gallon of water.
15. Carcasses of stock that die of rinderpest, black-quarter, haemorrhagic septicaemia, anthrax, pleuro-pneumonia and foot-and-mouth disease, should be buried and covered with at least six feet of earth. Put a lot of quicklime over the body.

16. The hides of cattle that die of these contagious diseases should be well scored and slashed with a knife and buried with the carcasses, to prevent their being used by the butchers.
17. The surface of earth floors of stalls and ground on which cattle affected with contagious disease have been kept should be removed and buried, and the earth below should be well dug up and turned over and the floor re-made with fresh earth. Brick and stone floors may be scraped, washed, and disinfected with quicklime, carbolic, acid or strong solution of phenyle.
18. Poles of carts and harness, or saddlery, etc., used by animals affected with contagious disease should be washed and disinfected. The old lining and stuffing of pack-saddles, etc., should be removed and burnt.
19. Mange in cattle and scab in sheep are both contagious, but are not of a fatal nature; still when these diseases are food among stock, the affected animals should be separated from the healthy and placed under medical treatment, to prevent the spread of the diseases and to cure the diseased animals as mangy cattle and scabby sheep will neither thrive nor fatten; moreover, some skin diseases are said to be inter-communicable from animal to man or vice versa.

Chapter 2

Some Common Complaints

There are some complaints among cattle, goats, and sheep that are common–that is to say, in large herd some of these complaints will always be present. They are simple ailments that can be easily cured, but, even in these simple diseases, great care and proper treatment by a veterinary surgeon are absolutely necessary. The least delay or neglect may result in something serious.

Cough

Sometimes cattle, goats, and sheep are troubled with a dry, hacking cough. Give a lot of young bamboo leaves every day, and give ½ chitak of ginger juice or juice of Bakash leaves mixed up with honey or treacle (*gurh*) every morning, and pot. or ammon. chloride 2 drams with honey every evening, until the animal is relieved. Half the quantity for small calves, goats, and sheep. Sometimes from ten drops to half a dram of turpentine or eucalyptus oil in from one to four ounces of unboiled linseed oil slightly warmed will prove very beneficial. Give the animal a lot of fresh green grass and warm gruel, night and morning for a week, and give half an ounce of condition powder twice a day, rub some warm mustard oil with some camphor, over the throat and sides and eucalyptus or turpentine steam for inhalation.

Weak Eyes or Watering Eyes

The eye must be well washed with one dram of alum or boracic acid and one pint of warm water three or four times a day.

Inflammation of the Eyes, or Ophthalmia

Causes

Blow from a stick or whip; dirt; insect or something in the eye; cold, damp, or excessive heat.

Symptoms

The eyelids are swollen; tears flow in abundance; there is great sensitiveness to light; the eye is bloodshot and covered with scum.

Treatment

Examine the eyes and remove all dirt and foreign bodies. Wash with a lotion of one pint of warm water to one dram of alum or boracic acid four times a day.

Give Epsom salt 8 ounces in 2 pints of warm water or 2 pounds of molasses and for small calves, goats, and sheep one to two ounces of castor oil in warm milk.

Keep the eye covered with a shade and the animal out of the sun and damp. Give nourishing and wholesome food.

Mange

This is an infectious disease.

Causes

Parasites in the skin, caused by ant of cleanliness, contagion, etc.

Treatment

Give the animal two ounces of salt and one ounce of sulphur with food every morning and evening for a fortnight, then stop the sulphur and continue the salt every morning. Give half a pound of Epsom salt in a quart of warm water once a week. Smaller doses for bigger calves, goats, and sheep; the smaller calves may be given a dose of castor oil (1 to 2 ounces).

Make a liniment of the following medicines and rub over the affected parts every morning:

Cocoanut oil	8 ounces
Spirits of turpentine	2 ounces
Gum camphor	2 ounces
Kerosene oil	1 ounce
Ground sulphur	4 ounces

The affected parts must be properly washed with hot water and soap and dried before the liniment is rubbed in.

Broken Horns

The horns of cattle, goats, and sheep are subject to accident.

Causes

Falls, blows, or struggles with each other in fights. The fracture bleeds most freely and may endanger the animal's life.

Symptoms

The injuries are of three kinds-

1st: The bone is broken, but the horn is not detached, and there is no open wound.

Treatment

Support the parts with a splint and bandage with adhesives, *e.g.*, plaster of Paris, starch, to keep them steady and at rest. The fracture will soon unite.

2nd: The horn is torn away and the bone is left bare and bleeding.

Treatment

First paint with tincture of iodine and tincture benzoine co., equal parts, and then over this apply Stockholm or common tar thinly and bandage the part with soft cloth and cotton-wool. The horn will not grow again, but the part will grow hard after some time.

3rd: Both the bone and the horn are snapped clean off, and there is a large open bleeding wound. Inflmmation or gangrene sets in.

Treatment

Immediately cut the broken remains of the horn to the level of the wound and bathe it with cold water and alum, or with tincture benzoin co. and the part bandaged with pressure until the bleeding stops; then dress the part daily with tincture of iodine and bandage.

Great care and cleanliness are necessary to prevent gangrene.

Leech in the Nose

Leeches often worry cattle, goats, and sheep by entering and fixing themselves in the nostrils while the animals are grazing.

Treatment

Inject a strong solution of salt water into the nostril, or else rub some dry salt on the part, and when the leech moves, draw it out with a pair of forceps or *chimtas*. Apply a little dry salt or alum to the part to stop the bleeding, or stop the drinking water for 24 hours: and after which allow it to drink, when the leeches will drop off after they are full with blood.

Wounds and Bruises

Wound and Bruises on cattle, goats, or sheep should never be neglected. They are liable to be troublesome and get infested with maggots.

Treatment

Wash with Condy's fluid or carbolic acid and water, or with phenyle and water, then dry up the parts and apply tincture of iodine and put a bandage round.

Enlarged Papillae of the Mouth

All ruminating animals have pointed papillae like points or thorns on the tongue and in the lining of their cheeks. This is caused by a disordered stomach or liver.

Symptoms

These papillae grow long and hard, and the cheeks, lip, and tongue of the animal grow tender, so that when the cow attempts to eat she is unable to do so. After a few days the mouth becomes yellow and furred and the breath smells very bad. A milking cow's milk will dry up.

Treatment

The mouth, tongue, and cheeks must be well rubbed with common salt or washed three or four times a day with a strong solution of salt and warm water to which add a few grains of permanganate of potash or in bad cases apply on the tongue and inside the mouth with some borax and honey.

Give the animal from half to one pound of Epsom salt with a pint of lukewarm water.

The animal must have plenty of rice or wheat gruel three times a day, with one ounce of salt in it each time.

If she will not drink the gruel, give it in a horn or bamboo *chonga*. Cattle that have sufficient salt regularly in their food are seldom troubled with this disease.

Wasting in Calves

Very often calves refuse their food or do not eat well; if neglected, they gradually become emaciated, and some severe illness follows. A calf will never refuse food if it be in good health, unless the food be dirty or otherwise unpleasant.

Loss of appetite is always a symptom of sickness. As soon as one finds a calf refuse its food, he should examine it carefully and see what is wrong. If no disease can be discovered, change its food; two drams of the condition powder every morning and evening. Two ounces of caster oil once or twice a week may be given.

If the symptoms continue in spite of the medicine, then it should be continued longer for a week or ten days.

If the symptoms be caused by worms in the stomach, then the treatment prescribed for worms to be adopted.

Cold or Catarrh

Calves and milch cows, sheep and goats, are often afflicted with this disease.

Causes

The disease is caused by exposure to draughts or wet, overcrowding in the house, dirty damp house, or not drying after bathing; also from infection.

Symptoms

The nose is dry, the eyes are watery, there is no discharge from the nostrils, the animal stands in one place as if stiff in the limbs, and does now chew her curd properly. There is more or less fever, and sometimes cough and purging.

Treatment

Immediately the sick animal should be separated. It requires to be immediately attended to, or it will end in some very dangerous illness. It is very frequent and fatal in calves. Juices from Bakash leaves and green ginger 1 ounce each mixed up with honey or molasses followed by a dose of Epsom salt 8 oz. (calves 2 ounces of castor oil), spt. Ammon. Arom. 1 ounce with gruel or water twice daily, may be given and the nostrils streamed with ol. eucalyptus or turpentine. When there is fever present 2 drams each of ammon. chlor and sot nitre in drinking water.

Should the discharge become thick and the nostrils and the eyes swollen then bicarbonate of soda 2 drams with tinct. squill or tinct. ipecac. one-ounce dose with water twice daily should be given (calves 1 to 2 drams) and the sides of the chest rubbed with mustard oil and camphor and ol. eucalyptus.

Accessory Treatment

Separate the animal from the rest and keep it warm and quiet. Cover it with a blanket and keep it in a warm but well-ventilated place. Wash the nostrils, eyes and mouth with permanganate and water.

No cold water must be given to the creature for twenty-four hours. Boil from two to four pounds of ground wheat and half a pound of linseed meal and give in a thick mash. When the animal begins to improve after twenty-four hours give it warm wheat or barley gruel to drink.

Sprains

The muscles or ligaments of the joints of the legs, muscles or tendons become ruptured or sprained due to a fall or some other injuries. The part swells and becomes hot and very painful and the animal is quite lame and may even be unable to move.

Treatment

As soon as detected the injured parts should be irrigated with cold water, or ice applied where available and cold water bandage put on and kept at rest, the bandage should be kept wet with a lotion of cold water and tincture of arnica or aconite. Goulard lotion soaked in a bandage may be applied. The part may also be fomented thoroughly, rubbed either with Elliman's embrocation or mustard oil and camphor or belladonna, or A. B. C. liniments.

Dislocation

Sometimes results from accident, over-exertion, a bone being put out of joint. It is a very painful thing and may terminate seriously if neglected for over such a short time. A veterinary surgeon should be called in at once.

Treatment

If no surgeon be available then the animal should be thrown down gently so as to have the dislocated joint uppermost and then the leg pulled and the part set.

The bone will be heard to return to its socket with a snap. After which rest and cold water and arnica application is all that is necessary. If there be much pain and swelling, one ounce of lead with tincture of arnica half an ounce in a pint of water may be applied to the part; or belladonna liniment applied twice a day. Elliman's embrocation is also good.

Sore Feet

Causes

Foreign bodies such as gravel, dirt, thorns, etc., in the cleft of the foot. If cattle are kept in wet and dirty places they will be troubled with sore feet.

Symptoms

Lameness, swelling of the posterns, pain. Matter forms and unless the object is let out and properly treated, ulcers form and become very troublesome and injurious.

Treatment

The feet to be carefully examined and all dirt and foreign matters that may be found removed; all dead hoofs to be pared properly. The feet should be washed with warm water and phenyle, and the matter if there be any let out. The part must be kept perfectly clean and after drying up, tincture of iodine and bandage applied and if no sore is present then wheat bran poultice applied with warm water and fixed by a gunny cloth.

Costiveness

Costiveness in cattle may terminate very seriously if neglected.

Causes

Dry, hard, coarse and unwholesome food, with insufficient drinking water.

Treatment

Eight to sixteen ounces of Epsom salt in a quart of warm water should be given; after 3 or 4 hours one pint of raw linseed oil-slightly warmed. An hour after, one or two quarts of thin warm rice-gruel, or water: Let it have no food until it is purged and afterwards only soft food in small quantities and one ounce of condition powder every morning for a week, with a liberal allowance of water.

Irregular Teeth

This is rare in cattle and is usually seen in the horse.

Symptoms

The beast eats less food than usual, and becomes gradually thinner and weaker; half-chewed food and saliva dribble from the mouth; the animal is tympanitic at times, and a bad smell issues from the mouth; the sides of the cheek and tongue are ulcerated, caused by the irregular teeth.

Treatment

The mouth must be carefully examined, and all long, irregular teeth must be shortened and smoothed by means of a tooth-rasp. If there be a decayed tooth or an abscess under the tooth, the tooth must be drawn out and the mouth washed with permanganate of potash and water, or salt and water, frequently.

The Naval Ill

Occasionally calves, kids, and lambs suffer from this disease.

Causes

Caused by the abrupt or imperfect separation of the navel cord, which makes the navel bleed; dirt, want of cleanliness and proper care; and infection. The house in which the calf is to be born must be thoroughly cleaned and disinfected and clean and dry straw put down.

Treatment

Immediately the calf is born, if the cord be of sufficient length, a ligature might be passed around the end and tied, and some tincture of iodine should be applied to it daily for a few days; but, if close to the abdomen, apply some iodine and methylated spirits, and then a little burnt alum with a piece of lint tied on to the part will suffice to stop the bleeding. Afterwards apply the following ointment: spirits of camphor, two drams; phenyle, quarter dram; pure vaseline, four drams; boracic powder, two drams; ground sulphur, one dram, after washing the navel with warm water and phenyle. The wound will soon heal.

If not attended to at once, an abscess may form in the part, and may lead to internal inflammation and cause death, or flies may blow the sore and breed maggots.

If an abscess form, follow the treatment prescribed for abscess. If maggots form, use the maggot destroyer and wash with a strong solution of phenyle and water.

Sore Teats

Causes

The calf nipping the nipples; leaving the nipples wet after milking; very hot or cold weather; want of cleanliness; injury from the nails of the milkers.

Symptoms

The nipples get chapped and inflamed; sometimes little pimples and sores form on the nipples; the cow becomes troublesome at milking, and kicks about; refuses to allow the calf to suck; the teats become very painful, and give forth a discharge which mingles with the milk; the milk lessens; inflammation of the udder may set in.

Treatment

Wash the teats well with warm water in which *neem* leaves have been boiled, or foment the part with hot water in which add some Epsom or common salt, then dry perfectly, and apply the following:

Vaseline, two ounces; spirits of camphor, one ounce; boracic powder, one ounce; mix together and apply morning and evening. Great care must be taken to gently draw out every drop of milk–if necessary, the teat-tube may, after boiling, be used carefully.

Preventive

Keep the teats clean and dry; rub some butter or mustard oil on them every time the cow is milked.

The Australian *Farm* and *Home* gives the following remedy:

For sore and cracked teats, wash with boric acid lotion. Boric acid is both cooling and healing, thus allaying inflammation and removing soreness promptly. It is also antiseptic in its nature, making its use a splendid thing from a sanitary point of view. Some dairymen require their milkers to wash their hands and the cow's udders in a weak solution of boric acid before each milking. The practice not only conduces to greater cleanliness, but absolutely prevents chapping roughness of teats and udder.

Chapter 3

Dangerous but not Contagious Diseases

Calving

Some cows have great trouble at the time of calving, and need proper medical treatment. If it be a cross-birth, or if the trouble be caused by contraction or deformity in the bone of the pelvis, or from tumors, dropsy, or the large size of the calf, the management will require professional knowledge and skill. Simple causes of the difficulty may be successfully overcome.

After-pains

After labour, if there be any pains, or to prevent any after-pains, tincture of arnica half to one ounce twice daily may be given for 2 days. Stop the food.

The after-birth or placenta, unless discharged soon after calving may also cause pain but there will be fever and general derangement. If it is not expelled by the cow within 4 or 5 hours, it will have to be removed by a veterinary surgeon and the uterus douched out with pot. permang. sol. or weak Lysol or phenyle sol. To hasten expulsion, paddy, barley (dry), and arrack 2 to 4 ounces with a pint of warm water, otherwise cleansing draught may be given. Bamboo leaves are also said to be very good. Warm gruel may be given.

Flooding

Allow the cow to lie down, and keep her quiet, with the hind parts rather higher than the fore. A bandage must be applied tightly round the belly and a cloth wet in cold water must be applied on to the vagina, quarters and over the loins. Injection of cold water may also be thrown up the fundament every half an hour.

The best medicines for flooding are ext. ergot. liq., or calcii lactate, 1 dram; adrenaline 1 dram is also very useful.

When the blood is black or brown and of a foetid smell, douching of the uterus with lysol sol. may be necessary until flooding stops.

Accessory Treatment

Great care must be taken to keep the cow quiet as rest is very essential.

Do nothing that will excite her. Do not force her to lie down. Do not force medicines down her throat. Give the medicine in a piece of bread or in her drinking water, or mixed up with some treacle.

Inflammation of the Womb (Metritis)

This usually occurs after the birth of a calf.

Cause

Undue retention of after-birth, difficult parturition, rough or dirty handling during delivery or removal of after-birth, use of dirty instruments, chill, slipping of the womb, and sometimes infection.

Symptoms

Constitutional disturbances, *viz.*, fever indicated by rough coat, hot mouth, horn and feet, dry muzzle, high-coloured urine, constipation, stoppage of food and rumination; severe straining either normally or during the passage of dung or urine; duty coloured offensive smelling discharge which is at first thin, then thick with shreds of membrane. The animal moves with difficulty, the back is slightly arched and in bad cases there may be slipping down of the womb or rectum as result of continued hard straining. There is generally great craving for water.

Treatment

Irrigate the inside with either weak lysol, phenyle or pot. permanganus twice daily, care being taken to see that the whole of the solution is removed by pumping. Internally cleansing draught with a dram of sodi sulphocarb. or carbo glycerine. The bowels should be kept open by laxatives and the strength of the patient kept up by one or two doses of stimluants such as arrack (country liquor), brandy or rum 2 ounces. The diet should consist of wheat bran, rice, sattoo or linseed gruel and green grass, etc. The animal should be protected from draught specially during winter sufficient bedding and water supplied.

Slipping Down of the Womb

Slipping Down of the Womb (Prolapsus Uterus and Vagina) is a common complaint with large, loose-limbed cows, especially if they are old, stall-fed with no exercise and have had many calves. Over-fat cows also suffer in this way. This is a complaint, more common among Mooltani and other heavy bred cows in Bengal than in other parts of India on account of relaxing climate, and if it is not attended to early, takes a serious turn and spoils the cow. The condition sometimes becomes chronic in which care should be taken to keep the animal in a place with the hind legs on a higher level than the fore; and if a cow is known to be liable to this trouble, it is not advisable to buy her at any price, however low.

Cause

The severe straining to expel the foetus; displacement of the womb; excess fat; irritation by hands or instruments when removing the after-birth or foetus, specially when they are dirty.

Symptoms

The womb is thrown out, and hangs between the hind-legs of the animal.

Treatment

This complaint wants particular care and attention. Immediately the womb slips it should be carefully washed with luke warm water, in which dissolve a few grams of permanganate of potash and then replaced, and chloral hydras ½ to one ounce dissolved in 2 pints of gruel given. No undue force should be used in attempts to replace the womb, but it should be gently and carefully pushed up by a process of gentle kneading till the whole is up into the pelvic cavity, and then it should be retained by the hand for a time, till the spasms begin to subside, when the hand may be gently drawn away. The vagina should be supported by a rope truss and the inside daily douched out with lysol. sol. (weak).

The cow must not be allowed to sit down, and she must be watched and not allowed to strain when in pain.

If not replaced at once the womb may mortify and the cow may also die.

If the services of an experienced doctor can be obtained, he should be immediately called.

Accessory Treatment

The cow must be kept perfectly quiet and confined to her stall, and have some warm rice or wheat gruel given her three times a day. No heating food should be given to the cow for a week or ten days.

Mammitis or Swollen Udder

Mammitis or Swollen Udder in milch cows is very serious symptom, and, if not taken in hand at once, may lead to much distress, and dry up the cow and may even prevent her from ever milking again.

Causes

It is a tendency to gathering caused by a chill by lying on a cold floor or a bruise, or some injury to the udder before or after calving, or by too high feeding before calving. If the cow is bathed, or her udder washed and not dried properly, her udder may swell. If there is a great secretion of milk before calving, and the milk is not extracted, it is likely to coagulate and cause inflammation. If the cow is not properly milked, and some milk is left in the udder, it may cause inflammation. Sometimes, giving the cow cold water to drink after she has calved causes it. If the calf bumps severely against the udder while sucking, it injures it.

Symptoms

One of the first signs of inflammation is the cow objecting to the bumping of the calf's nose. The udder is somewhat hot, red, swollen and painful; there is some difficulty in extracting the milk. Then little hard lumps can be felt in the teats or in some part of tile bag. The pulse is full, quick, and hard; the breathing quick and hard. The breathing quickens, the mouth and horns become hot, bowels are bound, and other symptoms of fever are present. If the disease is allowed to go on, the fever will become more severe; the cow will not eat or chew her curd; the hard swelling will become still harder in consequence of matter having formed; the milk will become curdled and mixed with matter and blood.

If the matter is not let out, it will spread through the udder, at the same time making its way slowly top the skin, through which it at last bursts, leaving deep long sinus. These heal with great difficulty, and in many cases portion of the udder or whole is lost. If this result is avoided, by judicious treatment, some hardening of the bag may nevertheless remain, which will take some time to remove.

Treatment

The ordinary treatment is as follows:

As soon as it is observed that the udder is swollen or painful, there is difficulty in extracting the milk, the affected parts should be thoroughly fomented with water boiled with *neem* leaves or Epsom or common salts about 2 pound mixed with one gallon of this water, after which the udder should be properly wiped and gently rubbed with the camphor liniment or warm bland oil and the calf allowed to suck in order to draw some of the inflammation. There is danger of the calf becoming ill by drinking the milk of an inflamed udder, so it is best to get the milk out of the udder by milking, or by means of the teat-tube or by gently drawing with the fingers. Give the cow from eight to sixteen ounces of Epsom salt in two or three pints of warm water, and keep her in a warm place. After four or five hours give eight ounces of raw linseed oil. If the bowels are not moved in twelve hours, repeat the dose. If available "Antiphlogistine" or other like stuff may be applied thickly over the affected udder and a suspensory bandage with some absorbent cotton-wool put on.

As soon as the least symptom of inflammation is detected, give internally tinct. aconite ½ to 1 drachm with two or four ounces of arrack if fever is present; foment; the affected part with boiled *neem* leaves, and gently rub the part with camphor liniment.

If the gathering softens, and points to an abscess, the matter must be let out with a lancet, and the wounds thoroughly washed out with warm water and phenyle, or a solution of tincture of iodine and water. Apply tincture of iodine and dust boracic powder and keep the udder bandaged and also provide necessary bedding (straw).

Accessory Treatment

The cow must be kept on simple food, as rice-gruel, wheat-bran and *doob* grass. Put salt in the food. The drinking water must not be cold, but luke warm. Rest and quiet are very necessary.

Preventive

If the udder fills with milk many days before the calf is born, extract the milk and empty the udder every morning and evening until the calf is born, then rub the whole udder with warm mustard oil with some powdered camphor in it. Immediately after the birth of the calf, draw out every drop of milk and rub the udder with the above oil. Also avoid the causes of the complaint.

Cure for Mastitis

Some drugs recently used in veterinary practice

J.N. Frost (*Coronel Vet.* 4, 1915, No.4, pp. 190-193)–The author states that during the year four herds in which infectious mastitis was spreading rapidly were treated with methylene blue. Each cow was given 60 grains followed by a dose of 30 grains the following night and morning. In all cases treated, the dose was sufficient to cause the milk to be coloured. Rapid recoveries followed in all the herds without the loss of a single quarter or the production of a hard milker. It is stated that one of these herds had been troubled nearly every year by infectious mastitis with the loss of the udder or a section of it, and the production of hard milkers by the formation of fibrous growths, commonly called spider, in the teat canal.

Treatment for Lumpy Milk

If the cow gives stringy or lumpy milk, the probability is that this is a case of mammitis or garget. There are several treatments for this, depending largely upon the cause. It might be caused from internal injury or from the cow lying on the cold ground. In such instances either hot or cold fomentations are excellent. Again it might be caused from feeding too much grain, or from the cow catching cold from exposure. In such cases half an ounce of saltpetre at a dose three times a day for three days in bran mash and followed by Epsom salt, one and one-half pounds at one dose dissolved in half gallon of water, is advised. Very often garget becomes a chronic disease, and when it does it is difficult to cure. If a cow becomes in this condition when she dries off again she ought to be disposed of.

Causes of Ropy Milk

A slight systematic derangement will cause this, the liver generally being the organ chiefly affected, but often in only such a comparatively mild degree that the animals give no visible signs of ill-health. Give a dose of Epsom salt, about ¾ lb., to each cow, and follow this up with a dose each alternate day of the following: bicarbonate of soda, one ounce; extract of taraxacum, four drams; extract of gentian, four drams; water, three pints. Dissolve the taraxacum and gentian with a pint and a half of hot water, and the bicarbonate of soda in the remaining one and a half pint. Mix the whole and give when sufficiently cool. There is usually some general cause, such as the existence in the food or water of some deleterious material which is the primary cause of this trouble. Allow the animal some salt with her food.

Rheumatism

The disease is rather common in some districts in India, especially in Bengal.

Cause

Is not yet thoroughly known. Exposure to wet and damp and draughts; damp floors, bad food, bad water generally aggravate the disease.

Symptoms

The animal becomes dull and droops and is disinclined to move. There is loss of appetite; pain in the joints and muscles, the pain shifts usually from one joint to another; one or more of the joints become inflamed and painful; the animal moves with difficulty; sometimes there is much fever. The complaint may last for only a few days, but is liable to return with change of weather.

Treatment

Sodii salicylate 2 drams with 4 drams of sodii bicarb. and 2 drams of pot. iodide with water twice daily is a very good remedy for rheumatism. Apply warm mustard oil with camphor or betul oil or old ghee to the affected parts. Or else the parts must be fomented three or four times a day with boiled *neem* leaves and Elliman's embrocation or lint A. B. C. rubbed in, and the joint bandaged.

Accessory Treatment

Place the animal in a warm and dry south room with plenty of clean dry straw on the floor and cover the animal with a blanket, and bandage the affected part with flannel. The creature should be fed on boiled wheat or gram, and *doob* grass.

Paralysis

Total or partial loss of sensibility and motion in one or more parts of the animal.

Causes

Injuries to the spine from blows; or in pack-bullocks from overloading; sudden changes of temperature and exposure to wet and cold or excessive heat. Some kinds of gram, *e.g.*, khesari, and herbs will cause it.

Symptoms

The animal staggers and drops its hind legs; loss of power in the limbs and inability to move freely. It falls and is unable to rise again; the pulse is full and slow, and loss of appetite; the bowels are bound, and the urine is retained, or the urine and dung are passed involuntarily. In severe cases there is inability to move the tail.

Treatment

Give powdered nux vom., ½ to 1 dram, with food twice daily. Foment the back and limbs with boiled water, and then rub A. B. C. liniment.

Accessory Treatment

Place the animal in a dry and warm room with lots of straw to lie upon. Turn her over twice a day, and give her a change of food. Great care and patience are needed, and feeding on boiled rice and wheat-bran and green grass essential.

Hoven

Tympany, distension of the first stomach or rumen with gas or wind. It is a common disease among cattle.

Causes

Irregular feeding; eating mouldy and bad food that the animal has not been accustomed to. Animals that have been almost starved for some time, when put into rich pasture or given grain, over-feed themselves, and the undissolved food undergoes fermentation and gas or wind is given off. Pasturing on marshy or inundated places, or eating fermented grass or food.

Symptoms

The symptoms appear suddenly and run their course rapidly. Swelling in the back portion of the left side of the belly, which, on being tappad with the fingers, is found to consist of wind in the first stomach; breathing is difficult; the animal neither eats nor chews the cud; the head is poked out; the animal grunts, stands quite stiffly, and appears unable to move; the eyes become red and thrust out of their sockets; the mouth is filled with frothy saliva, and the tongue hangs out of the mouth; the back is crouched, the legs drawn under the body. Should the animal lie down, the breathing becomes more difficult; the animal falls and struggles violently; sometimes sour fluid and food are discharged from the mouth and nostrils; lastly, death ensues.

This disease is very often mistaken for other diseases and is sometimes thought to be the effect of poison, on account of the very rapid way it runs its course. In acute cases the duration of the disease may be from one to three hours; in more protracted cases, the symptoms, may continue for twelve hours.

Treatment

Apply the "Express Mouth Gag" which removes the gas automatically and relieves the animal, or give internally one ounce each of turpentine oil and tinct. asafretida with 10 or 12 ounces of raw linseed oil, two doses at an interval of one or two hours. Foment the abdomen with hot water after an application of spt. or oil turpentine over the distended area. An enema of two quarts of warm water of 103° temperature with eight ounces of glycerine dissolved in it will relieve the animal. Wash the mouth with clean winter. If the case is severe, and after giving the above medicines no improvement takes place in a little while, then either the hollow probang or the trocar must be used, to remove the gas and to introduce medicines through the cannula of the trocar. The trocar must be plunged inward and downward into the paunch; through the left side of the stomach, midway between the last rib and the haunchbone. The cannula may be kept at the part for one or two hours if there be re-accumulation of gas.

Accessory Treatment

Until improvement, give no, food or drink. Give the animal thin rice gruel and, little soft green grass and plenty of salt for a few days after improvement sets in. Also give one or two pints of linseed oil or 8 ounces of Epsom salt with 2 pints of lukewarm water for 2 or 3 days followed by half an ounce of condition powder every day.

Grain Sick

Impaction of the rumen or first stomach with food, either of a coarse or tough and indigestible kind, such as over-ripe wooloo-grass, weeds or uncooked whole grain.

Causes

Indigestible and coarse grass or weeds; unground and uncooked or unsteeped grain; too large a quantity of food; insufficient supply of drinking-water. When the stomach is overloaded, it becomes at first torpid in action, and from the continued pressure and distension of its muscular coat it ceases to act on account of the latter becoming powerless.

Symptoms

The symptoms are somewhat like those in hoven. In hoven the stomach is filled with gas; the left flank, on pressure, feels soft, elastic, and yielding to the fingers; on percussion, it sounds hollow and drum-like; frequent belching; the wind that escapes has an offensive smell; respiration quick, short, and pulling; position standing, head stretched forward, unable to move; moans, and appears in great distress; eyes red and staring. In grain-sick the stomach is packed with food. The symptoms appear gradually. The animal is dull and does not chew the cud; the left flank gradually swells, and, when tapped with the finger or pressed on, is hard and pits as if pressing on soft earth. The bowels are inclined to be constipated; the animal generally keeps standing; fluid is sometimes discharged from the mouth and nose; the animal grinds its teeth and grunts. As the contents of the stomach ferment, the stomach becomes more distended; the pulse becomes weak and small, the respiration becomes more difficult. Death is caused from suffocation. The disease lasts from one to three days.

Treatment

Give the animal one pound of raw linseed oil and then give nux vom. powder one dram with about ½ lb. of Epsom salt and repeat this or oil after 2 or 3 hours. If the animal seems to be in much pain, then before giving it nux vom. give liq. ammon. fort., 4 drams, in linseed oil, two doses at an interval of fifteen minutes. An enema of two quarts of hot water and eight ounces of glycerine should be given if the bowels continue very much bound. Foment the abdomen and push on 2 ounces of country liquor every 3 or 4 hours. If inflammation of the stomach follows, give tinct. belladonna, 4 drams, every 3 to 4 hours. Inflammation is recognized more or less by pressure on the distended stomach giving the animal pain.

When the medicines fail to act, and the symptoms increase in severity, the stomach must be relieved by cutting it open and taking out the contents by a veterinary surgeon.

This operation requires a practised hand.

Accessory Treatment

The animal must have nothing but rice, linseed and barley gruel for two or three days, after which, small quantities of fresh young *doob* grass should be given in addition to the gruel. Give the animal plenty of salt and pure drinking-water. Also give one ounce of the condition powder every day for a week.

Preventive

Give the animal soft food in moderate quantities; give abundance of pure drinking-water at least three times a day. Hard and dry substances should not be allowed. Food should not be given in very large quantities or too frequently.

Fardel-Bound

Impaction of the third stomach with hard, dry, and indigestible food, which accumulates and becomes so very hard, dry, and caked between the folds or leaves of the stomach as to always arrest more or less its functions, and in severe cases to cause total obstruction. This is also a very serious condition and when detected should at once be placed in the hands of a competent veterinary surgeon.

Causes

This disease occurs more frequently in the hot season, and is common in a season when there is an unusual scarcity of pasture and water. Cattle and sheep are then driven from sheer hunger to eat hard and fibrous grasses and weeds, or branches of shrubs and trees, and the third stomach is unable to grind down such bard and unwholesome fodder, and the latter gradually accumulates, hardens, and cakes within the stomach.

Symptoms

The animal does not chew the cud; there is a loss of appetite; respiration is quickened, and is accompanied by a grunt, not unlike the grunt which is heard in pleuro-pneumonia. The bowels are constipated, sometimes at the commencement there is slight diarrhoea, but, as a rule, there is constipation; now and then, a small amount of liquid faeces, with very hard and dark-coloured pieces of the caked fodder, detached from the leaves of the third stomach, is passed; the urine is high coloured and not unfrequently there are signs of hoven.

If relief is not afforded, inflammation of the stomach sets in. In that case the respiration becomes increased and the grunting more audible. The animal grinds its teeth, and its countenance is peculiarly expressive of pain; the mouth, ears, and horns become cold, the pulse very small and thready, and numbers from eighty-five to a hundred. Any dung passed is partly liquid and partly in small hard cakes and very offensive. The grunt now becomes a moan. Sometimes, in the last stage the animal will be in a state of stupor; in some cases symptoms of great excitement occur, and these probably depend upon the fourth stomach having become inflamed. The duration of the disease is from five to fifteen days.

Treatment

The treatment must be with the view to relieving the overloaded and impacted stomach of its hard, dry, and caked contents.

Give the animal Epsom salt from four to eight ounces in a pint of hot water, or half a pint of raw linseed oil with half a pint of warm water, two doses at an interval of one or two hours and foment the stomach. The salts and oil may be given in conjunction with tinct. or pulv. nux vom. (4 and 2 drams} and pulv. ginger ½ ounce.

To keep up the strength of the animal, ruin or arrack 2 ounces may be given with rice gruel daily.

Accessory Treatment

Give the creature plenty of thin warm barley gruel at short intervals during the day and night.

This will assist much in opening the bowels and in softening the caked food in the third stomach and facilitating its escape. Very often many days elapse before all the hard stuff is got rid of; therefore it is necessary to continue giving the gruel until no hard caked pieces are found in the dung. After the animal has recovered give it soft green grass in small quantities.

Preventive

Soft and easily digestible food, abundance of drinking-water, and regular supply of salt.

Choking

Choking is the obstruction of the food pipe and as a result there is inability to swallow.

Cause

This condition may be caused by hard and large pieces of food, such as mango-seed, onion, potatoes, turnips, carrots, etc., becoming lodged in the back part of the throat or in any part of the gullet–the channel by which the food passes from the mouth to the stomach.

Sometimes foreign bodies, such as pieces of leather, bone, iron, nails, sharp thorns, sharp pieces of wood, etc., are taken by cattle and become lodged in the gullet, and when very hard, with sharp edges or points; may lacerate the lining membrane of the tube.

Symptoms

If the obstruction is in the back part of the mouth or throat, the animal coughs and salivates, and when drinking, the water will be returned by the nostrils.

If in the gullet, after making two or three swallows and filling the gullet as far as the point of obstruction, the water will be returned by the mouth and nostrils.

The animal is very uneasy; his countenance shows signs of pain; spasm or cramp of the muscles of the neck will be observed. These are owing to the animal endeavouring to make the lodged body go down to the stomach, or to be returned by the mouth. In a little time signs of hoven appear, and if the animal be not soon relieved, the left side of the belly will become much swollen.

If the obstruction is in the throat, by introducing the hand into the very back part of the mouth it will be felt.

If it is in that part of the gullet between the back part of the mouth and the chest, it will be felt on the outside, as there will be a swelling at the point of obstruction. There may occasionally be certain amount of difficulty in breathing.

If it is lodged in that part of the gullet which passes through the chest, then the negative evidence of its not being found in the back part of the mouth, or any part of the throat, will be conclusive, and when the animal drinks, water will be observed passing down the gullet along the lower part of the throat without meeting with any impediment; but after the animal has taken two or three swallows the gullet, at the throat portion, will gradually become filled with the water, until at last, when quite filled up to its junction with the throat, vomition of it will occur.

Treatment

Give very carefully and gradually warm linseed oil half a pint, with arrack two ounces, well mixed together.

This will lubricate the gullet as well as the impacted food or foreign body, and stimulate the gullet to act and force it onward.

The medicine may be returned by vomition once or oftener, but it must be perseveringly given and again and only a little at a time and gently.

If the cause of obstruction is lodged in the throat, it must be removed by the hand; if in the back of the throat portion of the gullet, after giving the oil and arrack press with the fingers all round the swelling observed in the neck, and it will very often be thus moved a little, then give a little more of the oil and arrack, and again apply more pressure to the swelling; and by so persevering the impacted body will generally pass onwards, and the animal will be relieved.

If by the symptoms it is evident that the part of the gullet within the chest or at the neck is obstructed, and the steady perseverance in giving the oil and arrack has failed to remove it, then a hollow elastic tube, if at hand, may be introduced by the mouth down the gullet to the part obstructed, and a little gentle pressure will generally move the cause of obstruction onwards to the stomach. If a proper tube is not to be obtained, then a good rattan cane, about the thickness of the forefinger, with a soft ball of cotton or tow about the size of an egg, covered with cloth, and securely fastened around the one end of the cane, may, after being well soaked in oil, be introduced by the mouth into the gullet, and pressed gently against the impacted body. During this operation the mouth must, be kept open by an assistant.

It now and then happens that the gullet is cut or torn by the impacted body, or by the operator using too much force with the tube, or from the ball not being properly fastened on the end of the rattan cane, and thus the gullet may become permanently injured, and in such a case choking is very apt to recur. It is always advisable to secure the help of a veterinary surgeon from the beginning,

Whenever choking happens, the part of the gullet obstructed will remain weak for some days, so only soft food, such as gruel or mashes, must be given for three or four days, and afterwards young green grass.

Opening the neck portion of the gullet, in extreme cases, may be necessary when the obstruction is in that part.

Red-Water

Tick-fever or Bovine Malaria. This is a blood disease, resulting from the invasion of the red cells of the blood by a parasite and the consequent faulty preparation of the blood, etc., and the blood becomes thin and weak.

It is accompanied with fever, red coloration of urine, much prostration and debility and in severe cases with emaciation. Only cattle are liable to the disease; more frequently cows are attacked, especially a short time after parturition, and probably this depends upon the shock to the system by the parturition.

Causes

It is caused by a parasite. Some undrained low-lying lands are known to yield pasture giving shelter to ticks which transmit the disease. The pasture may be very rank, non-nutritious, or bare, and mixed with acrid herbage. It has been proved that when such lands are properly drained, manured, and cultivated cattle pasturing them cease to suffer from red-water.

The disease very often attacks the cattle of 3 months and upwards but young calves are practically immune and one attack confers a great degree of immunity, and cattle bred upon infected farms are more resistant, spring and autumn months are favourable for the disease.

The disease is common in India and the continent.

Symptoms

This appears in acute and mild forms; the acute form is sudden in its onset and frequently fatal. The animal is very dull, keeps away from the herd, there is profuse salivation, groans, arches its back, grinds its teeth and often staggers and falls. Skin is dry and there is almost always a profuse watery and violent diarrhoea, the temperature goes up to 107°F, difficult respiration, membranes pale, and after a day or two alarming symptoms may subside, and there is change of coloration (reddish-brownish or blackish) of the urine. In milch cows the milk decreases and may be pinkish. Sometimes lung symptoms supervene and death follows. In the chronic or mild form the symptoms are less marked and sometimes passed unnoticed. Death is not very common and recovery takes place after a week or 10 days.

The animal becomes very weak; the lining membranes of the mouth and eyelids are pale in colour; the eyes are sunk; the mouth, ears, and legs cold; the pulse very weak; respiration rapid; the animal lies down much, loses-condition rapidly, and soon becomes emaciated. Signs of abdominal pain are frequent; the animal becomes very weak, and is unable to rise; death ensues in some cases.

The duration of the disease is from 3 to 8 days.

Treatment

Cattle can be immunized against by inoculation of blood from recovered animal and if it severely reacts it should be controlled by subcutaneous injection of trypanblue 100 c.c. of a 1 per cent solution in water–the inoculated animal remains a carrier of the disease for the rest of his life and is a source of danger, so it should not be allowed to be introduced into a clean area.

The eradication of the disease is bound up with eradication of ticks which can be done by successful occasional dippings of the affected animal in some arsenical preparations, and by burning the grass of places known to be favoured when riot in the animal's body.

Accessory Treatment

Abundance of good wheat and barley gruel must be given frequently, and the animal kept in a dry and warm place.

Preventive

Good pasturage, regular supply of salt and drinking-water, proper shelter and protection against ticks.

As soon as a case occurs in the herd, it should be placed in the hands of a veterinary surgeon.

Indigestion and Diarrhoea

This disease consists in frequent purging, generally without fever or constitutional disturbance; but sometimes with signs of abdominal pain. The frequent and inordinate passing of watery dung results from a disordered state of the stomach and bowels.

Causes

It generally arises from the animal having taken some unwholesome forage, acrid herbage, or foul water. Indigestion is frequently the case of diarrhoea.

The herbage grown on certain lands produces it, and very often such lands are marshy and badly drained. In the Punjab it is known by the name of *chooknee*, and has of late years attacked the cattle of that province in seasons when pasturage and water were scarce, and the animals were obliged to eat unwholesome herbage and acrid shrubs and drink very foul water.

An over-dose of purgative medicine may also cause diarrhoea. Again, in cases where the stomach and bowels become over-loaded, diarrhoea may follow.

In rinderpest, haemorrhagic septicaemia, the last stages of pleuro-pneumonia and other blood diseases, looseness of the bowels invariably appears. This is also a symptom in arsenic and other poisoning. Cold or sudden chill has been known to produce it, especially when the bowels have been in an unhealthy condition. Exposure to great heat is sometimes another cause. It may also be caused by dirty contaminated food or unclear feeding vessels.

Diarrhoea generally attacks herds when grazing on lands yielding the first shoots of green grass after the first fall of the rains.

Symptoms

A frequent passing of watery dung with or without offensive smell; at first with no straining or pain.

The appetite generally remains good; the acumination may be a little irregular, and the secretion of milk may also be less than usual; but the general health of the animal seems but little affected.

If the purging continues long, then there will be straining at the time of passing dung and the back will be arched; more or less pain will be shown, and sometimes blood will be passed with the dung. Ordinarily it is Nature's effort to get rid of the poison from the system.

If it continues long, the animal becomes very much emaciated and weak.

Treatment

Give the animal a pint of linseed oil. If there be any pain, flatulence or blood in the motions, give linseed oil with turpentine oil ½ ounce mixed up with gruel. Half the quantity for calves, sheep and goats. Do not check the diarrhoea at once; if it continues more than four or five hours, then give medicine.

When the diarrhoea is persistent then give bhang (Indian hemp) ½ tola or opium 30 to 60 grs. in a pint of oil.

Acid sulphuric dil., 2 drams, or astringent powders may also be given with rice gruel, if the diarrhoea continues for one or two days.

When the colour of the dung is either black or clay and the smell from it is offensive, give acid nitro-hydrochloric dil. half to one dram, with a pint of chiretta water twice daily, for a few days.

Accessory Treatment

Clean water, and barley, *jaw-sutto* mixed with hot water and allowed to cool, arrow-root gruel, barley or rice cooked with one or two green chopped bael fruit may, after straining through a cloth, be given with advantage. After the diarrhoea has stopped, give the animal a dram of the condition powder twice a day, and feed on wheat and barley gruel and soft sweet *doob* grass for a few days.

Epilepsy

Causes

Young, well-fed, fat cattle and more frequently the calves are the most liable to it. Exposure to the sun in the hot weather and over-exertion on a hot day will aggravate it. Sometimes the intestinal worms are, also said to be the cause of this affection. The calves of stall-fed cows without much exercise are most susceptible to this condition.

Symptoms

The beast staggers and falls suddenly; often bellows in the most alarming manner; every part of the body is violently convulsed; the tail is lashed, the teeth are ground, the mouth closed, and the jaws fastened together; the breathing is quick, and attended with heaving at the flanks; frothy saliva dribbles from the mouth, and the power to retain urine and dung is lost. The convulsions become gradually less severe, then they cease, and the animal seems as if nothing had happened out of the usual way.

Treatment

During the fit, make the animal inhale some smelling salt or carb. of ammonia and bathe the face and head with cold water. Nothing more can be done during the fits but as one attack is apt to be followed by others, the treatment must aim at their prevention and cure. Give the animal tinct. belladonna (cows, 4 drams; calves, m. x to m. xv), or pot. bromide (cows, 2 drams; calves, gr. x to gr. xv) morning and evening. Fits are apt to recur at regular intervals or periodically. A little while before such times the medicines should be given at intervals of one hour.

If worm is suspected give thymol or santonine, 5 grs., or juice from, pineapple leaves, etc., followed by a dose of linseed or castor oil.

The bowels should always be kept open.

Sometimes nux vom., powdered or tincture, gives satisfactory result.

Apoplexy

Causes

Sudden rush of blood to the head, followed by effusion of blood on the brain, producing pressure and terminating in some lesion of the blood-vessels, caused by excessive heat and over-exertion, or over-feeding.

Symptom

Sudden insensibility with loss of sensation and motion. The attack is sudden, but the premonitory symptoms are-general listlessness, and indisposition to motion; breathing, low and somewhat laboured; slight fulness and protrusion of the eyeballs. When the animal is struck down, the breathing becomes stertorous, slow, and laboured; the pulse is full and slow; frothy mucus issues from the mouth; the skin becomes cold, eyes glassy, bowels torpid; struggles violently for a time, and dies.

The animal may linger for from one to twenty-four hours.

Treatment

Apply ice over the head and neck if available, otherwise pour cold water from a height on the head and back for some time, and give the following remedies.

If from heat, give tinct. belladonna, ½ to 1 ounce, or chloral hydras, ½ to 1 ounce, mixed up with little molasses or honey every 2 or 3 hours until consciousness returns.

If from over-feeding, give tinct. nux vom. ½ to 1 dram, in the same way as the above.

Give an enema of two to four pints of hot water and eight ounces of glycerine. The abdomen may also be fomented; sometimes a removal of a quantity of blood gives satisfactory results. A veterinary surgeon should be consulted at once.

Accessory Treatment

The animal will remain weak for some time, and must be fed only on gruel and a little soft grass. Quiet and rest in a shady place are very necessary.

An animal once attacked will always be very susceptible to the sun and heat.

Inflammation of the Brain

Causes

Fracture of the horn; blow on the skull; hydatids bladder-worm, in the brain.

Symptoms

Dullness and heaviness; eyes staring and congested; hurried respiration; full and slow pulse; sometimes very restless and the animal rushes at everyone before it, and gallops about with raised tail and arched neck; tears up the soil with its horns and feet; bellows; at last it tumbles down quite exhausted.

Treatment

It is best to put the case in the hand of a veterinary surgeon at once; apply ice or cold water over the head and spine.

Give it the following remedies:-tincture aconite and belladonna 3 to 6 drams every two hours will also be helpful. Give the animal eight ounces of Epsom salt in a quart of warm water if possible. Hot water enemas are also helpful.

Not many animals recover from this disease.

Accessory Treatment

Nothing but thin gruel should be given to the animal until the symptoms abate.

Colic or Gripes (Pain in the Abdomen)

It is more common in horses than in the cattle.

Causes

Cold; chill; rotten food; uncooked, unground, or over-steeped grain; tough grass; bad water, etc.

Symptoms

Pain in the stomach, indicated by uneasiness and restlessness; pawing the ground; striking the stomach with the hind-legs or horns; frequent getting up and lying down; grinding the teeth, moaning, etc. If it arises from the presence of wind in the stomach a swelling will be observed in the stomach on the left side; the wind will pass from the fundament and the mouth.

Treatment

Give a dose or two of the following mixture: 2 drams of asafoetida and a pint of linseed oil, after which give Epsom salt 8 or 12 ounces with some ginger juice in 2 pints of warm water twice daily for one or two days for a clearance.

The following mixture may also be given with advantage: brandy, four ounces; black salt, one ounce; powdered ginger, one ounce; Bishop's seed (*ujwain*), two ounces; camphor (gum), twenty grains; and linseed oil from eight to sixteen ounces. Mix well and give in one dose. From a quarter to half the quantity for calves, goats, and sheep. Ten minutes after this medicine has been given, give the animal a quart of hot water to drink.

Cows seldom get colic, but half-grown bulls often do.

Accessory Treatment

A man should be set to hand rub the whole of the abdomen unless the cow is in the advanced stage of pregnancy, when rubbing must not be resorted to, specially the right side.

Give the animal only warm wheat or rice gruel, and no other food for a day or two. Plenty of salt is necessary in the food.

Preventive

Avoid the causes.

Parasitic Warbles

This name designates a disease which occurs specially in warm weather and is caused by the gadfly sitting upon the skin of the cow's back for the purpose of depositing one or more of its eggs. These eggs are licked up by the animal and pierce through the food-pipe and go under the skin and undergo a change and gradually develop. The result of this is a small swelling, which the insect of the hatched egg occupies until the following hot weather or rains, when it makes its escape, or when this swelling is lanced or even pressed hard the insect comes out and falls on the ground and in a short time becomes a fly on its own account, propagating the species by the same process that begot itself. There may, of course, be numerous swellings upon the cow's back, and each is the temporary habitation of the gadfly.

They sometimes very seriously injure the general health and condition of the animal, and invariably injure the hide by riddling it with holes, and cause considerable commercial loss and great irritation to the animal.

The following is an extract from an English paper:

"The bot-fly, or warble-fly, is a very widespread pest and inflicts great suffering and injury on the animals affected by it. The parent-insect lays its eggs just in the upper surface of the skin, and the infant grub at once tunnels inwards. Once well established underneath the hide, it makes a sort of chamber, where it lives its course, keeping the unlucky beast in which it dwells in a state of constant irritation and annoyance. The result is to set up an inflammation round the cell, which sometimes extends over a large surface on the animal's back. Sometimes there are evident signs of general illness, which, in very severe cases, may even lead to death; but, in the vast majority of instances, the only sign is the habit the animal indulges in of licking the affected place. In these cases the havoc wrought is not apparent until after slaughtering, when the hide reveals on its underside hollow pits, which open into holes in process of tanning. The carcase, more-over, is injured by the inflammation, which is the true cause of what butchers know as 'licked beef.' It is estimated that from one-quarter to one-third of the beasts which come to market in England are thus affected, to the great loss of the breeder and all concerned."

Although the disease is not very fatal yet it entails heavy commercial loss.

An instance is quoted in which 102,877 hides were passed through a market in twelve months and 60,000 of them were warbled.

The loss on these hides alone is put down at £15,000.

Treatment

Lay hold of the swelling between the finger and the thumb arid squeeze it out and inject tincture of iodine or spirits of camphor into the hole with a small syringe. This will thoroughly destroy the grub, and prevent many other cows from being affected by the insect.

Hydatids (Bladder-worms)

These are generally found in the lungs or liver, sometimes in the brain, consisting of a sac lined by a thin bladder or cyst filled with a limpid colourless fluid; in this a number of cysts, from the size of a pea to a child's head or even bigger are found imbedded in the tissues.

Causes

Hydatids are caused from grazing in infected pastures by dog's stool as the parasites remain in the intestine of a dog. The disease shows itself generally after the monsoon weather when pasturage is not drained properly.

Symptoms

The presence of the disease cannot be ascertained, but may be suspected from the following symptoms: loss of appetite; suspension of rumination, dry muzzle, hot ears and horns, hurried breathing; rough staring coat; rapid emaciation; sometimes there is no indication of disease except loss of flesh or hairs, diarrhoea, difficulty in breathing and general wasting.

Treatment

Give the animal half a pound of rock salt (*Sundhub lobon*), pounded and dissolved in two quarts of warm water, with two ounces of powdered sulphur added to it, in the morning, for a couple of days. After that give two ounces of the salt every morning for a few weeks. Dimol is considered by some to be very good. Consult a veterinary surgeon.

Accessory Treatment

Give the animal plenty of good wholesome food and salt and pure water. The house should be clean, dry and sweet.

Inflammation of the Bowels (Enteritis)

This is more common to horses than cattle.

Causes

Cold, chills, bad food and water, acrid substances, poisons.

Symptoms

Fever with shivering, thirst, hard and frequent pulse; the pain in the abdomen which becomes so severe that the animal tumbles down, turns its eyes about, and throws its head from side to side as if in great agony; the horns, ears, mouth, and feet become cold; breathing hurried; eyes very red; the animal will not allow its stomach to be touched; diarrhoea and mortification of the bowels sets in; death ensues.

Treatment

At the commencement, tinct. aconite is indispensable; give every 2 to 3 hours; then give tinct. belladonna every two hours. Also give from 8 to 16 ounces of unboiled linseed oil or olive oil. The stomach should be fomented with blankets, out of which hot water has been wrung.

Stimulants, *e.g.*, brandy, rum or country liquor, may also be necessary.

An enema of two pints of hot water and eight ounces of glycerine should be given. It is advisable to consult a veterinary surgeon.

Accessory Treatment

Keep the animal out of the draught, and give it only barley or thin warm gruel.

Hernia

Hernia is displacement of organs from their natural position and usually appears in both acute and chronic forms.

For the proper treatment of this disease you need the services of a veterinary surgeon.

Jaundice

Jaundice is a symptom of disease generally affecting the liver, and not a disease itself. In which all the visible mucous membranes and even the skin become yellow. Consult a veterinary surgeon.

Poisoning

Cattle die from poisons either accidentally taken with their food, or criminally given to them.

The poison may be either vegetable or mineral.

In parts of India cattle are poisoned by *chamars* (butchers) so that they may obtain their hides. It is the custom generally throughout India to throw the carcasses of cattle that die on the waste land (*bhagar*), and the hides are considered the perquisites of the *chamars* of the village. In some districts *chamars* pay a rent to the zemindar for the right of taking the hides.

Chamars sell most of the hides to hide-merchants, and in many districts an agreement between the *chamars* and a hide-merchant is drawn up and signed, whereby the hide-merchant agrees to give so much money for a certain number of hides, provided they are supplied by the *chamars* in a given time; and it is customary for the hide-merchant to give some money in advance to the *chamars*.

This often leads to the *chamars* poisoning cattle in order to obtain a sufficient number of hides by the time mentioned in the agreement;

and they have often been detected, either in giving the poison by their own hands to cattle; or employing their agents or wives and children to administer it.

The common mode adopted is to mix the dose of poisons with a little *ghee* or flour, put on a plantain or other leaf, and put it into the mouth of the animal or throw it on the ground in front when feeding, for him to eat up.

Another plan is to scatter the poison over a sweet bit of pasturage.

The third plan is to introduce the poison with a sharp instrument through the skin into any part of the body.

The poison commonly used is one of the preparations of arsenic, either white or yellow, generally the former; sometimes vegetable poisons, such as jequirity, *dhatura*, aconite, *madar*, and nux vomica are made use of.

It is believed that arsenic is sometimes provided by the hide-merchant's agents, and given to the *chamars*.

Poisoning is probably often extensively carried on under the cloak of outbreaks, that is, when rinderpest is prevailing in a district, more hides are secured by poisoning. Again, the *chamars* are well aware of the contagious nature of rinderpest, and an instance has been recorded of their having taken the contents of the stomachs and bowels of the cattle that had died of the disease to a distant village where the epidemic had not prevailed, to scatter over the pasture-lands there, in order that the disease might be contracted by the cattle of the village, and they might have a new source of obtaining hides.

Cattle are sometimes poisoned by eating the *"castor oil plant and seeds,"* and in seasons of droughts, when pasturage is scarce, from eating acrid plants and herbage.

Symptoms

When poisons are eaten by or given to a bullock or cow in large doses, the symptoms are as follows: the animal becomes suddenly ill; is seized with a trembling fit; has most severe abdominal pain; strikes the belly with the hind-legs or horns, and looks frequently round to the flanks; foams at the mouth; has great thirst; very often shows tetanic twitchings; shows signs of hovea; passes dung very often; diarrhoea sets in, and with it more or less blood is passed;

generally, in from two to four hours death occurs, the time depending in a great measure upon the amount and kind of poison administered.

Treatment

The dose of poison generally given is so large that treatment is seldom of use, and the antidotes are not at the hand of the cattle-owners.

But if detected in time, the following treatment may save the animal. Two quarts (or *seers*) of sweet oil (olive oil) or pure unboiled linseed oil poured down the animal's throat. Repeat the dose after an hour, or moist peroxide of iron freshly made in repeated doses.*

Accessory Treatment

The diet should be linseed gruel, bran mash, ishapgul soaked in water and boiled rice; but no grass or straw should be given for two or three days, after which soft *doob* grass may be allowed.

Abscess

When an abscess forms on the udder, face, foot, or any other part of the cow's body, foment the part with boiled *neem* leaves and apply tinct. iodine or emp. belladonna fluid. This should be done twice or three times a day. Or else the belladonna liniment should be applied, and when possible a linseed poultice put on the part. The poultice should be changed 4 or 5 times a day, the part may also be blistered with bin-iodide of mercury ointment (1-8) to hasten suppuration.

When ready, the abscess should be opened and the pus let out; after which it should be properly washed with phenyle and water and dressed with tincture of iodine and gauze. It should be properly dressed twice a day, and the part covered up by a bandage if possible, to avoid its being fly-blown.

* This is made by adding carbonate of soda or sol. of ammonia to tinct. ferri. perchlor. and the resulting precipitate filtered through a handkerchief, or by dipping a red-hot iron in water, or, if handy, ordinary iron-rust may be given dissolved in water.

Chapter 4

Contagious and Fatal Diseases

Rinderpast (Cattle-Plague)

Names: Boshonto (Bengali), gootee, matah (Hindi), etc.

Rinderpest is a contagious fever of a typhoid type. It is the most fatal and contagious disease known in cattle. Under ordinary treatment, from 20 to 50 per cent of the plain cattle attacked die, but the mortality is much higher (about 90 per cent) among the hill and imported animals, *viz.*, English, Australian, etc.

Causes

Unknown contagion: the time that elapses before an animal shows symptoms of the disease, after being exposed to contagion, is generally short, being from three to eight days; but sometimes it appears in as short a time as twenty-four hours.

Symptoms

The first symptom is increased temperature of the body; but this can only be tested by the use of a thermometer. The symptoms to be noticed by keen observers may be divided into three stages:

First Stage

Dullness; shivering fit; coat staring; mouth hot; mucous lining of the mouth congested; short husky cough; ears drooping; bowels generally constipated, and the dung coated with mucus; appetite partially lost; thirst often great; spasmodic twitchings of the muscles of the body, especially of the back, shoulders, or hind quarters; back arched, and the four legs drawn together; rumination slow and irregular; grinding of teeth; yawning; tenderness of the spine; pulse accelerated, keeps away from the herd.

Second Stage

Mouth, ears, horns, legs, and other parts of the body vary in temperature, being at one time hot, at another cold; respiration is much quickened; appetite lost; rumination ceases; slight discharge from eyes; increased tenderness of spine; keeps away from other animals in the herd or lies down, with head turned back to the flank; fever high; thirst great; difficulty in swallowing; twitchings of muscles more marked; pulse very quick, but irregular; difficulty in moving; gums and buccal membrane and papillae very red, afterwards small pinhead-like white spots appear in them; tongue furred; bowels very costive; the pellets of dung coated with mucus and blood and then gradually become loose (semi-solid); lining membrane of rectum and vagina very red and dry; tenesmus; and occasionally prolapsus of rectum and vagina.

Third Stage

Profuse discharge of very viscid mucus from eyes, nostrils, and mouth; very offensive breath, excoriations, coated more or less with white aphthae, of gums, corners of the mouth, buccal papillae, and roof and floor of the mouth and tongue, also sometimes inside the nostrils and eyelids; purging now sets in, the dung at first consisting of small hard pellets, covered sometimes with blood and mucus, and watery faeces, and afterwards of fluid matter only with flakes of mucus, blood, and aphthae, and is most offensive and fishy in odour; the temperature comes down; occasionally gas-filled swelling under the skin. Great prostration; continued thirst, but greater difficulty in swallowing, followed by coughing, coldness of skin, horns, ears, legs and mouth. Cows in calf generally abort. The animal lies down, indeed has no power to rise; moans, breathes with difficulty, grunts; liquid greenish yellow and sometimes bloody faeces are involuntarily passed, the pulse is imperceptible, and death generally occurs in two to six days. Sometimes an eruption of the skin is seen about the dewlap, udder, groins, shoulders and ribs; but this eruption is not by any means an invariable symptom, and when it occurs, it is generally found in animals attacked in the hot season. This eruption is considered a favourable symptom, as, when it is profuse, dysenteric symptoms seldom prevail, and recovery often follows; when no eruption on the skin occurs, and violent dysenteric symptoms continue, death generally ensues.

The disease is not improperly considered by some cattle-owners to be a kind of pox. It is called *natah* by them when the eruption of the skin is evident, and is described as *andar-ka-matah* when the lining membrane of the stomach and bowels is so much affected as to lead to the passing of blood, mucus, and aphthae.

In some cases, especially in those of imported and English cattle which run rapid course, symptoms of high fever and congestion of the mucous membrane of the mouth and delirium are shown by the animal becoming excited, and after plunging about, it will fall down, and become insensible and die.

If a cow is in calf, unless very great care is taken, she will slip her calf. Sometimes even with the greatest care this mishap cannot be prevented.

Treatment

In India, treatment is often successful and this may be attributed to the disease very often appearing in a mild form. Rinderpest belongs to a poisonous material contained in the system must gain exit to allow to the patient recovering. The chief aim of the treatment should be to aid nature in ridding the system of the poisonous matter, and to support the strength of the animal by good care, nursing, and proper diet.

Ordinary Treatment

Immediately the first symptoms appear, give the animal pot. permang., 2 drams; arrack, 2 ounces in a quart of warm gruel or water, and repeat the dose every 4 or 5 hours.

When purging and passing of blood and mucus continue for more than twenty-four hours, the following draught has proved successful:

Powdered gallnut or gallic acid	2 drams
Powdered catechu	2 drams
Powdered chalk	2 drams
Arrack (country liquor)	4 ounces
Water	2 pints
or mixed up with rice gruel	

This should be repeated every 5 or 6 hours until the purging ceases.

For sheep and goats, one-sixth of the above dose should be given.

Indrajab and ishapgul, ½ tola each, powdered and soaked in ½ gallon of water mixed with little sugar should be given twice daily as drink.

Indigenous Treatment

Fresh roots of the *chirchery* plant, two ounces; fresh leaves and roots of the *jokha* plant, two ounces; thorns of the *shimul cotton* tree, two ounces. Have the whole pounded or ground together very fine. dive a dose of twenty to forty grains of this medicine in rice gruel three times a day for three days.

Ten grains for a dose to a calf, and five grains to a goat or sheep. All villagers know the first and last-mentioned plant and tree, but *jokha* is the *Santali* name for a plant that grows wild in their district. The Bengali name of the plant is *jogabalta*, and the Hindi name is *jukkha*.

Homoeopathic Treatment

As soon as the first symptoms are seen, give aconitum nap. lx, and arsenicum alb. lx, ten drops alternately, every three hours; when the eruption appears, give antimonium tart. lx, one grain, every three hours. If the eruption is driven in, give spirits of camphor, ten to twenty-drop doses, every ten or fifteen minutes, until the skin gets warm and the eruption reappears. Sulphur 3x is very good when the eruption is disappearing and there is great itching, etc.

If possible, a veterinary surgeon should be called in.

Accessory Measures

Immediately remove the sick animal from the rest of the herd. Until purging sets in, as much *cold* water as the animal will drink should be allowed it; but when purging sets in, give *cold* water in small quantities. The diet must consist of rice and wheat or barley gruel, well boiled with chopped green bael fruits (2 or 3) and of good consistency. Cool well, strain in a piece of cloth, and give one or two quarts three times a day. Nothing hot or warm must be given. Put some salt in the gruel. When the animal begins to get well, give it some fresh *doob* grass besides the gruel. Hard, dry, fibrous food must, on no account, be given; for some weeks after the creature has recovered. It may cause serious illness.

The mouth of the animal should be washed with a little warm water and pot. permang. It must be kept in a house, or room, free from draughts, but plenty of fresh air must be allowed the creature, and the room must be well ventilated. Nothing is of so much importance as unlimited supply of pure air and water.

If the skin seems very painful, sponge the whole surface with warm water with a few drops of carbolic acid, or water in which *neem* leaves have been boiled and some ground turmeric has been dissolved. If the cow is in milk and the calf is let to drink the milk, the poor little thing is sure to get the disease.

The milk must be regularly extracted and buried. If the milk is not extracted from the cow, her udder will become very painful, and she will be in great distress. If there are eruptions in the udder and teats, some butter or camphorated or boro-vaseline may be applied; and if the part is inflamed, it should be fomented with phenyle water and then the above ointment applied.

All the dung and soiled litter must be immediately removed and burned and buried, and the place kept perfectly clean.

Sprinkle some pure carbolic acid or phenyle with hot water or lime about the room.

Preventive

The disease arises from contagion. Never let the cattle graze on the public roadside or run with outside cattle, or allow any outsider to come to the cattle shed.

When the disease is prevailing in the district, have all the healthy cattle inoculated with anti-serum by a veterinary surgeon immediately.

Foot and Mouth Disease

The disease is known by different names in different parts of India. The most common names are, *khoori, khurrah, khoorpocha* and *aesho* (Bengali).

It is a highly contagious fever, accompanied with vesicular eruption in the mouth and feet and on the udder. Sometimes the mouth only is affected, at other times only the feet. In some cases the feet become first affected, in others the mouth.

It attacks cattle, sheep, goats, pigs, and fowls; and even man has become affected from drinking the milk of cows suffering from the disease.

It is constantly prevailing more or less in all parts of India, and the country cattle usually get the disease in a very mild form, but the English and other imported and heavy-bodied animals suffer badly. The calves are very susceptible and the percentage of death is much greater in them, as they often die of exhaustion.

An animal may suffer several times during its life from this disease.

Causes

In the majority of cases the disease is caused by unknown contagion, but it may be spontaneous in its origin, and is probably due to the animal having been kept in a stall or ground in a filthy state.

Very often it is difficult to trace the cause, but it is scarcely ever found where cattle are kept in a clean state and by themselves, that is, not allowed to mix with other cattle or frequent highways; so the cause would generally appear to be due to contagion and want of cleanliness.

Experience proves that the period of incubation is from twenty-four hours to three or four days, out generally thirty-six hours.

Symptoms

The symptoms first noticed are a shivering fit followed by fever, lameness in some cases, hot, mouth, horns, and extremities, with smacking of lips, and frothy salivation. Then, vesicular eruptions will be noticed in the mouth and feet and in cows, on the udder and teats. The eruption is like blisters of the size of a bean or more. These vesicles or blisters are sometimes seen on the nasal membrane; they burst in eighteen or twenty-four hours, and leave red sore spots, which either soon heal or turn into ulcers.

The tongue is chiefly affected, but the gums, dental pads and roof of the mouth and the inside of the cheeks are, in some cases, also affected.

The eruption in the feet will be found at the junction of the skin with the hoofs, and between the hoofs.

From the mouth and feet being very sore, and the existing fever, the animal does not feed, and is very lame on the feet affected, the animal shaking the hind limb in the air.

If the animal be a bullock and be kept at work, the symptoms will become more severe, the legs will swell, and very often the hoofs will be cast, and sometimes abscesses will form. in the legs.

When the eruption is on the udder and teats, there will be swelling and tenderness of both.

If the milk of an affected cow be drunk by the calf or by man, they will become infected.

In milch cows, the teats often become very sore from the blistered parts being pinched by the hands of the milkman, and the udder sometimes swells and becomes inflamed from the milk not being drawn away.

The hands which milk diseased udders will carry the contagion to the udders of sound cows, if care is not taken to well wash the hands after milking an affected cow.

Goats and sheep are similarly attacked, but suffer in the feet most; when sheep and goats are afflicted, they get much out of condition.

The disease is sometimes mistaken for rinderpest, but in foot-and-mouth disease, as found in India, purging is not one of its symptoms, whereas diarrhoea and dysentery are invariable accompaniments of rinderpest. Again, in rinderpest the feet are not affected.

It is possible for an animal to have at the same time both rinderpest and foot-and-mouth disease, but such a case is rarely met with.

If an affected animal is properly cared for, all symptoms of fever will disappear in three or four days, and the animal will be well in ten or fifteen days with little loss of condition; but care is not taken of the animal, and in the case of bullocks, if made to work, the fever will become severe, the appetite, less, and from the ulceration extending between the hoofs and the feet, the hoofs may drop off the legs will become much swollen, and abscesses will form in them, death occurring in ten or twelve days.

When the cattle are large and heavy, they suffer more from this disease than lighter and smaller ones.

In some attacks the disease is mild, in others, of a severe type.

In India, the percentage of deaths among those, attacked ought not to exceed two or three per cent, and with common care an animal rarely dies from this disease.

Ordinary Treatment

Wash out the mouth two or three times a day with a quart of warm water, to which add five grains of permanganate of potash or two quarts of warm water in which dissolve twelve ounces of common salt or 2 ounces of borax or alum.

Wash and foment the feet with phenyle and warm water and soap, twice a day, carefully removing all dirt especially from between the hoofs, and dress the sores with either tar (Stockholm), 4 parts, and phenyle, 1 part, or with the following dressing oil and bandages applied.

Mustard oil	8 ounces
Turpentine	4 ounces
Camphor	4 ounces
Phenyle	1 ounce

The udder, teats, and other parts affected with sores should be kept clean and dressed frequently with tie above-mentioned dressing, which will prevent flies blowing the sores and breeding maggots. If the flies attack the mouth, then camphorated oil should be applied to the mouth twice a day. The udder and teats may also be applied with boro-vaseline or camphorated vaseline (1-8) or hot ghee or butter.

When there is much fever, give the following twice a day:

Ammon. chlor.	3 tolas
Camphor.	¼ tola
Nitrate of potash	3 tolas
Arrack	½ chittack
Water	4 chittacks

As soon as the least sign of the disease is discovered, separate the animal from others.

Wash the mouth and feet as directed.

Accessory Measures

The animal must be kept housed and clean, and the floor of the house must be kept scrupulously clean, and the house or room thoroughly ventilated. Give the animal plenty of fresh air.

Doob, or some soft green grass and rice gruel, with an ounce of salt and three ounces of treacle, must be given to the creature twice or three times a day.

Sprinkle pure carbolic acid and water or phenyle and water about the room.

Preventive

The disease, in the majority of castes, arises from contagion. Adopt measures recommended in Chapter 1.

Malignant Sore-Throat (Haemorrhagic Septicaemia)

Galaphula (Bengal), Ghararwa (U.P.), Galghotu (Punjab), Avroe (Mumbai). This is a fatal and very contagious disease. Calves are very liable to get it. It occurs during the rains and animals remaining in low-lying lands are most subject to this.

Causes

Blood-poison, caused by a micro-organism, from impure air and water; contaminated food; wound-infection; bad feeding; bad housing (*see* Chapter 1).

Symptoms

The first symptoms often are those of influenza; loss of appetite; suspension of rumination; cough; discharge from the nose and mouth and eyes; fever; inflammation of the lining of the nostrils and eyelids; swelling of the throat and glands below the ears and between the jaws; swelling of the tongue and the back part of the mouth; difficulty in swallowing and breathing; profuse salivation; breath becomes very noisy and offensive; diarrhoea; the tongue protrudes from the mouth and is dark in colour, ulcerated, and has purple patches on some parts. The head is protruded, and there is great weakness.

The symptoms rapidly increase, and the animal dies from suffocation in from one to two hours, or two or three days.

Treatment

The course of the disease being very rapid, treatment is either of no avail or impossible. If the animal be taken in hand early, at once separate it from the others, and try the following treatment. This disease is almost similar in character to diphtheria. Give carbo-glycerine 1 dram or acid salicylas 2 drams with gruel, or treacle twice daily, or alternately, every three or four hours. Wash the mouth and nose with permanganate of potash and water frequently.

An injection, at the seat of swelling, of a 10 per cent carbolic solution may also be given and also warm water enemas medicated with carbolic acid, every half an hour, may be beneficial.

Accessory Treatment

The house and everything connected with the animal must be kept perfectly clean. Barley, wheat, or corn gruel must be given to the animal in small quantities frequently; a tablespoonful or a small wineglassful of brandy or country liquor (arrack) must be given with the gruel, if there be extreme weakness. A hot bath may do the animal much good, but a blanket must be kept over it after the bath. Free ventilation in the room and cold water to drink are very necessary.

In any case the doctor will have to be called to take up the treatment immediately. The meat, skin, urine, and dung of the diseased animal are very poisonous, and all should be buried.

The healthy animals of the herd should be protected by inoculation of anti-serum immediately.

Bronchitis

This is a very dangerous disease, and is sometimes infectious.

Causes

Exposure to wet or cold, or to sudden changes of temperature; a neglected cold or catarrh; or contagion.

Symptoms

The symptoms at first are those of a common cold, and afterwards seem to be similar to those of sore-throat; the cough at first is very dry and has a grating sound; there is a mucus discharge from the nose and the mouth; the cough becomes very painful and frequent; the countenance appears anxious and distressed; the breathing is quick and heaving and obstructed, in consequence of accumulation of tough, tenacious phlegm; there is unwillingness to move; the breath is hot; the cough is increased by moving about; no food is eaten; the animal wastes, and the skin becomes dry and bound to the ribs; coat stares and looks unhealthy; death ensues. It may end in inflammation of the lungs (pneumonia).

Treatment

The animal must be kept in a warm but well-ventilated room. Give tinct. aconite 4 drams, arrack 2 ounces mixed up with honey every 5 to 6 hours.

When there is inflammtion of the eyelids, and a discharge from the eyes and nose of a watery kind, give steam inhalations of oil eucalyptus or turpentine through the nostrils.

When the discharge from the eyes and nose is of a mattery character, and the supply of milk is scanty, give tinct. squill or ipecac. ½ to 1 ounce with treacle and 2 ounces of arrack twice daily.

The following liniment must be well rubbed into the throat, chest, and sides:

Mustard oil	8 ounces
Spirits of turpentine	8 ounces
Camphor of turpentine	2 ounces

In severe cases the chest must be plastered with mustard and flannel bandage or antiphlogistine or the like stuff applied.

Accessory Treatment

Keep the animal perfectly clean and warm and quiet. Give it wheat, barley, or corn gruel, in small quantities (one pint of quart) frequently. The gruel should be warm.

Water should be given in small quantities occasionally.

No grass, straw, or leaves must be given for some days.

Bronchitis from Worms

This also is a very dangerous and infectious disease. Calves and yearlings, and young goats and sheep, are specially subject to it.

Causes

Small worms of a silvery white colour in the windpipe and its branches, caused by impure water and food, or insufficient supply of pure water; worms in the water, grass, or grain; impure air; over-crowding. If one animal is affected, then many more of the same herd will be attacked, if preventive measures are not adopted.

Symptoms

There is a slight discharge from the nostrils and a dry, husky cough, which becomes most violent and comes on in fits; the animal is dull and drooping, and quickly loses flesh; there is much distress in the chest, and the animal grunts often; goats and sheep cry out as it in great pain; a thin discharge flows from the nose; loss of appetite; great weakness; as the disease increases, the symptoms become more severe, and death follows in a few weeks.

Treatment

Loss of time and neglect of the premonitory symptoms will prove fatal. The only thing to be done is to detach and expel the worms. This may be done by one of the following remedies:

1. Pour one teaspoonful of chloroform down each nostril of the animal; a less quantity must be given to smaller animals.

   This treatment has proved successful in many cases.
2. Mix thoroughly, and give every second or third day. Half the quantity for small calves, goats, and sheep.

Creosote	1 dram
Turpentine	2 drams
Spirits of camphor	½ ounce
Linseed oil	4 ounces

Accessory Treatment

The affected animal must have one ounce of sulphur and two ounces of salt every day in its morning and evening food, or with a little gruel before its food. It should have lots of gruel and bran mash, but dry, hard food should not be allowed.

The affected animal must be separated from the rest, and the nostrils steamed with creosote, turpentine or eucalyptus, sulphur may also be burned in the room, so that it can inhale the fumes.

Preventive

Cleanliness in food and drink; regular, supply of salt and sulphur in the food; sufficient food and water; separation from the affected ones.

Black-Quarter (Called Black-leg or Quarter-ill)

This is a blood disease, and is contagious and fatal. It is generally accompanied with a swelling under some part of the skin, generally on the loins, or hind or fore quarters, neck and abdominal wall. The swelling is puffy and crackles when pressed upon by the hand, as if blown out with air.

The disease has been found to appear very suddenly.

Causes

Is due to a special bacillus which gains inside the system through wounds. The younger cattle between the ages of 6 months and two years are specially liable to become affected, as in them blood is more, rapidly formed than in older animals. The most thriving animals are the most susceptible, especially those which are rapidly improving after having been in somewhat low condition.

In certain badly drained lands in Great Britain, the disease was wont to occur frequently; but since the lands have been properly drained, the disease is seldom met with. In some parts of the continent of Europe and India, the disease is always more or less present at certain seasons, on lands where the drainage is defective.

Doubtless in India, outbreaks of black-quarter frequently depend upon cattle pasturing on marshy lands.

When one head of a herd is attacked, it is a most certain that others will also become affected, not merely from contagion, but also on account of having been probably fed and cared for in a manner similar to the one ill.

Symptoms

The attack is generally very sudden. An animal, seen perfectly well a short time before, may be found in an hour or two afterwards to be dull, stiff, and lame which will attract the attention and shortly after swelling will be observed under the skin in some part of the body, generally on the loins, hind quarters, fore quarters, and rarely on the throat and tongue. Sometimes the disease may be located in the chest or abdomen.

When the swelling under the skin is examined, it is found to crackle under the pressure of the fingers, and to feel as if blown out with air; this is owing to gas being generated by the causative organism, and when the skin of the part is cut open it emits a very nasty smell, and the muscles are seen to become blackish, then the breathing will be distressed.

The disease, though sudden, may be preceded by dullness and listlessness. The patient refuses food, but may be thirsty at first and drink greedily; there is fever, rumination ceases; the ears, horns, and muzzle are hot and dry; breathing is hurried, with expanded nostrils and open mouth; breath hot; flanks heaving; and constant moaning is observed. The pulse, full and excited at first, becomes weak, and tremulous; subsequently, the animal is disinclined to move; the neck and head are extended; eyes protrude and are congested; the animal may become unconscious or insensible; when induced to move, it staggers and is lame in both hind quarters, constantly drooping on either to obtain ease; it tumbles down and makes vain efforts to rise. These symptoms increase in severity, and the animal dies of exhaustion in twelve, eighteen, or twenty-four hours.

Treatment

Is useless, but it is recommended that susceptible animals may be inoculated one month before the onset of the season when outbreaks are known to occur.

Another treatment is to give the animal internally forty drops of tincture of iodine in four ounces of water three times a day, and apply and inject tincture of iodine to the swelling.

Wash the mouth with cold water constantly.

Accessory Treatment

Keep the animal wall sheltered and give it lots of pure water to drink; mix eight ounces of common salt and four ounces of Epsom salt in a quart of water twice a day. Give it no food for a day or so; on the second day only thin gruel should be given. Barley gruel is the best.

Preventive

When one of a herd is attacked, others will have a tendency to become affected; it is, therefore, advisable to adopt preventive measures. Give the animals from two to four ounces of Epsom salt and the same quantity of common salt dissolved in water, morning and evening, for three days, and plenty of pure cold water to drink. Protect them from sudden changes of weather. Keep them on bare grass, green, soft, and fresh.

The lands must be properly drained, and dirt and offensive matter at once removed from near the place.

Preventive inoculations may also be done.

Dysentery

Inflammation of the lining membrane of the large intestines, sometimes accompanied with ulceration. It is usually seen in young calves and may also be contagious.

Causes

Neglected diarrhoea; eating unwholesome grass or plants; drinking bad water; exposure to severe cold or damp at night, or excessive heat in the day; feeding upon marshy or badly drained lands; overwork; want of good and sufficient food; contagion. It is sometimes due to intestinal worms and also eating oilcakes and other foods in excess.

Symptoms

Skin hot; dullness; anxiety; hair slightly rough; uneasiness; pain in the abdomen; straining; passing blood and mucus with the dung; the animal wastes, and loses appetite and spirits; sometimes the dung is dry and in small lumps, but generally the discharge is watery and attended with severe pain; the rectum may become everted; sometimes the skin and mouth become yellow; the animal wastes away.

Treatment

Give the animal hail a pint of raw linseed oil with 2 drams of oil turpentine and then give castor oil emulsion in small doses every 4 hours. Keep a blanket round the stomach and abdomen. If the purging be excessive, give decoction of kurchi bark and salt solution enema and afterwards astringent mixture for calves.

Accessory Treatment

Give arrowroot or barley gruel, boiled with green bael (chopped up). It must be given in small quantities–a pint for a large cow-frequently. Give one quart of ishapgul (½ tola soaked in 2 pints of water) twice a day. When the dung hardens give rice and linseed gruel. No grass or leaves must be given for some time. Keep the animal clean and dry and in a clean, dry and well-ventilated house; if the night be cold, put a blanket over the animal. The abdomen should also be wrapped round with cotton-wool and bandage.

Slinking or Abortion

Bringing forth the calf before the proper time. The cow generally slinks between the fifth and eighth month after conceiving. Abortion is sometimes contagious.

Causes

Blows, falls, strains, jumps, severe exertion, forcible movements, and other injuries; rinderpest; hoven; internal inflammation; high fever; eating certain herbs that grow on marshy or badly drained lands; drinking dirty water or water impregnated with iron; intercourse with the bull during pregnancy; exposure to bad smells, arising from rotten matter, especially if it be the cleansing of a cow that has just slinked-the cow is said to abort from "sympathy"; over-feeding during pregnancy, over-heating food or insufficient food; fright and contagion.

Symptoms

One has to be very observant to notice the symptoms that warn of the approach of the mishap. Unless proper means are adopted at the first appearance of danger, there is no chance–of averting it. The symptoms are: dullness; loss of spirits; want of appetite; loss of cud; hollow flanks; enlargement of the lower part of the belly; disinclination to move; unsteady walk; the calf does not move at the flanks; breathing laboured; a yellowish discharge from the vagina; the belly continues to fall; fever sets in; the animal moans; the calf is expelled at last. It is either already dead or lives only a short time. In most cases abortion occurs without much premonitory symptoms and usually a dead calf is seen lying in the stall next morning although nothing was the matter with the animal the previous evening.

Treatment

If the discharge from the vagina is foetid, then it is sure the calf is dead, and the sooner it is expelled, the better.

If the calf is alive, do all you can to prevent the miscarriage. Give anodyne draught (chloral hydras or pot. brom.) every six hours. Pour cold water over the loins and haunch and keep the animal quiet, preferably in a dark room.

If there is discharge of blood, have the inside irrigated with Condy's fluid or weak phenyle or lysol solution. When the abortion is caused by blows, falls, and injuries, give anodyne draught to allay pain.

Accessory Treatment

Remove the cow from the others, arid keep her quiet in a clean and well-ventilated room. Give her light and sloppy food, and pure cold water. The dead calf and the after-birth and every trace of the abortion must be either burned or buried deep underground far from the other cows.

Cow-pox (Variola)

This is a contagious disease, but is not fatal, and usually runs a very mild nature except in cases of gross neglect. It is an eruptive fever and attacks animals generally only once in a lifetime.

Cause

Generally, infection.

Symptoms

Eruptions about the centre and base of the teats and sometimes on the udder itself in the form of circular pustules, which, when fully formed, attain the size of a four-anna bit. The disease may show itself and run its course, followed by some constitutional disturbance without detection, except in the instance of milch cows.

The pustules are generally situated on the udder and teats, and irritate milch cows so that they become restless and violent during the process of milking. The pustules are of a circular form, with its centre depressed and margins raised and filled with a clear fluid, which gradually becomes opaque and purulent, and is surrounded by a red blush of inflammation. In the course of a few days the pustules burst and scabs form; the scabs dry und fall off in fortnight or three weeks. In most cases it passes off unnoticed with few red pimples and is taken for mosquito bites and the pustules, when formed, break by the hand of the milker which soon heal up. Sometimes the udder swells up very much and is painful; the cow will not allow the calf to suck, nor will she allow herself to be milked. Unless care is taken to milk, the milk will dry up and the cow will. be spoiled. Sometimes the animal has small lumps all over her, and under her skin, they are so soft as not to be felt by the hand, but they give the coat a rough, lumpy look.

Treatment

Separate the animal at once. Wash the affected parts with *warm* water in which dissolve a few grains of permanganate of potash, and smear with fresh butter or *ghee*, to which add a little *neem* oil or boracic powder or camphor powder. Every drop of milk must be extracted. If there be any difficulty in doing this, then tie the cow's hind-legs together, and foment the udder with warm water and permanganate of potash; do not make the water very hot, or else you will injure the udder. When the udder becomes soft, wipe it dry with a clean dry cloth, and rub it over with butter or ghee and boracic. Then commence to milk her, but be careful not to press the fingers on the pustlues. Thus you may extract all the milk. The cow must be treated with great tenderness and care.

Accessory Treatment

Keep the animal in a clean, dry and thoroughly ventilated room, and feed it on light, sloppy food. Withhold everything indigestible.

Milk Fever or Parturient Apoplexy or Dropping after Calving

It is a very dangerous and infectious disease. It generally attacks the best and heavy milch cows, and that more than 75 per cent. of the cows attacked die.

Causes

Unknown, but is now believed to be due to deficiency of calcium salts in the system.

Symptoms

The disease generally shows itself from the third to the fifth day after calving. Sometimes the disease begins on the first day. The cow refuses her food, or eats very little of it; she is depressed, hangs her head, and looks dull; the horns are hot; the nose is hot and dry; the urine is scanty; bowels are confined, or the dung is hard and lumpy; the pulse is quick and full; the breathing is quickened, and the flanks heave. In the *second stage* the milk is reduced or nearly stopped; the eyes glisten, and look bright and staring; the white of the eye is covered with red streaks, or it is of a leaden colour; the cow looks anxious and weak; the hind-legs seems weak and are set apart from each other; she is restless and uneasy; she does not chew the cud; all discharge from the bearing is stopped; the calf is neglected; the pulse becomes slow, and the breathing more difficult; the udder sometimes becomes hard and swollen, and there is great difficulty in drawing out the milk. *In the third stage* the cow gets startled; the breathing becomes more hurried, and the flanks heave much; the mouth opens, and saliva flows from it; the animal staggers and falls, the body begins to swell, the extremities grow cold; there is shivering; with cold perspiration; she struggles, as if in great pain; death ensues.

Cows with their third or fourth calves should be carefully observed after calving, especially if they are deep milkers, as at this period they are very apt to develop milk fever. If a cow is lying down with her head tuned into her side, you should go to her and place her head in a different position. If she persists in returning into the old position again, you may suspect that she has milk fever.

Treatment

The classic treatment is inflation of the mammae with sterilized air after stripping the milk off. The gland should be massaged to distribute the air.

If the stomach is distended either have it tapped or the new "express" mouth opener applied, or tube passed and the rectum and bladder relieved; the animal drenched with stimulants and laxative if it can swallow, otherwise injected.

Carefully watch the newly calved cows during the first 12 hours and at once seek veterinary advice if warning symptoms appear.

Modern treatment of calcium chloride sol. injection may be adopted.

Every drop of milk must be extracted three or four times a day. The calf should not be allowed to drink the milk. Consult a veterinary surgeon.

Accessory Treatment

Keep the cow in a dry, cool, and thoroughly ventilated room; the open air is preferable to a closed room, if it is dry and warm. If the body is very hot throw a blanket over her. Give her some warm rice, wheat or barley gruel, three or four times a day, also warm water to drink.

No grass or other food should be allowed until the symptoms subside. Keep the room and the animal perfectly clean. Wash the vagina two or three times a day with warm water and permanganate of potash. If the discharge from the vagina smells bad, inject some Condy's fluid and warm water into it.

Preventive

The disease is contagious. The likely animals should be fed upon sparing diet of laxative food for a week or 10 days before they are due to calve and to allow them gentle exercise, and small amount of milk, should be withdrawn during the first 6 or 8 hours after calving and at intervals and gentle massage of the udder after each milking.

When two or more cows calve at the same time or within a week of each other, keep them apart. Keep newly calved cows away from the affected animal. Avoid the causes mentioned above. Wash the vagina with permanganate of potash and warm water. If a cow is subject to it, give her a dose of Epsom salt in warm water, twenty-four hours after calving.

White Scours in Calves

Is a contagious disease affecting calves within the first 3 weeks of life, in which the chief symptoms are severe whitish diarrhoea, great dullness, progressive emaciation and weakness, and death usually occurs in 3 to 10 days.

Cause

Bacterial infection, possibly through the unclosed navel, unclean and insanitary stable and overfeeding and unclean and unwholesome milk, etc., predisposes the disease.

Symptoms

Sometimes it commences very early, even a few hours after birth. There is profuse yellowish or greyish white diarrhoea with offensive smell, the temperature rises at first, but later comes down. There is great dullness and emaciation, arching of the back and, due to continued soiling of the back, tail and abdomen with dung, blisters appear over the part of the skin.

Treatment

Mostly preventive-disinfect the stall, and hind parts of the cow before calving, and strict antiseptic precaution in treating the navel with tincture of iodine as soon as the calf is born and providing clean bedding, etc.

Curative-is very doubtful, common scours may be treated by cutting down the feed one half and giving four drops of formalin to each quart of milk–allowing the calf to drink small quantities of lime water will sometimes cure scours, the following mixture may also be given: sodii bicarb., 2 parts, bismuth carb., 2 parts, hexamine, 2 parts, barley or rice water boiled-give one ounce with 4 ounces of milk every 3 or 4 hours.

Cases of all scours at the Wisconsin College of Agriculture are treated as follows, according to a news report from that institution:

As soon as symptoms appear, two or four tablespoonfuls of castor oil are mixed wich one-half pint of milk and given to the calf. This is followed in four to six hours by one teaspoonful. of a mixture or one part salol and two parts subnitrate of bismuth. This dose can also be given with one-half pint of new milk, or the powder can be placed on the tongue and washed down by a small amount of milk. The ingredients named can be obtained at any drug store and mixed in the proper proportions at the time of purchase.

Calf Scours

A successful dairyman says–"I think I have the best remedy for calf scours I ever heard of, and it may be useful to some of your readers. I put from one teaspoon to two tablespoonfuls of ground ginger in the milk, depending upon the age of the calf and conditions. In addition, I always cut down the quantity of feed one-third to one-half, and begin with a small dose. This increases the hunger of the calf and makes him less particular, while the smaller feeds are better for the disordered stomach."

Scours in Calves

The Kentucky Equipment Station has used very successfully the following drugs in the treatment of scours for the last eight years, during which time not a single calf has been lost from scours, although approximately twenty calves have been born each year.

If the calf is developing a case of scours, it is taken in hand immediately, placed in a clean stall, well bedded, and given a dose of two ounces of castor oil, one tablespoonful of Listerine, and one teaspoonful of Paregoric (tinct. camphor co.). All these ingredients are mixed thoroughly, put in a long-necked bottle, and given to the calf with some milk in the form of a drench.

The dose repeated in six hours if necessary.

If the case is severe, ten drops of laudanum or acid sulph. dil. are mixed with the above ingredients.

Calves, three or four months of age, are often cured by giving three ounces of castor oil.

In bad cases the diet should consist of only barley water or barley boiled with few pieces of chopped green bael fruit and water and strained in a piece of cloth.

Worms in the Intestines

There are three principal varieties of parasites that invade the intestines of cattle, goats, and sheep. There may be more than the three kinds mentioned, but these three are the principal ones.

They are (1) the small thread-worm; (2) the long round-worm; (3) the tape-worm. The thread-worm is generally from a quarter to one inch or longer, of a silvery white colour, and often exists in clusters or balls chiefly.

The long round-worm is very much like the common earth-worm, but nearly white, and measures from about six inches to one foot or more. They usually never exist alone.

The tape-worm often exists alone, and measures from three inches to many yards in length.

The thread-worm and the long round-worm in the same animal at the same time, are found to exist is also the long round-worm and the tape-worm in the same bowels. The calves are the worst sufferers.

Causes

Impure water and food. Worms in the water and food often cause the disease. Young calves suffer from it when they are over-fed with milk; swallowing flies will cause it. Infection: If one animal in the herd or flock has got worms, the rest are likely to be infected also. The worms are swallowed in the food.

Symptoms

The only certain proof of the presence of worms is the detection of them, or their ova, in the dung, or in what is thrown out when the animal coughs. But the following are some of the symptoms noticed in the infected animal: A short, dry cough; eating or licking of mud; diarrhoea; loss of appetite; rough, staring coat; dropping of the ears; grinding the teeth; pain in the stomach; wasting; passing of slime, and blood and sometimes worms and sometimes rubbing the buttock and nose against the wall or floor. In calves, often epileptic fits are noticed.

Treatment

Immediately you detect the least symptoms of worms in the intestines, give the animal the following:

Spirits of turpentine	1 dram
Spirits of camphor	80 drops
Castor oil	2 ounces

Mix the whole thoroughly, and pour it down the throat gently. The dose should be repeated every four days or week, until the worms die and are passed out in the dung. Stop the above medicine and give two to four ounces of Epsom salt in a pint of warm water, early in the morning, and keep it tied up for an hour; if during that time it is not purged, then give it a dose (four to six ounces to calves and one pint to cows) of linseed oil. Repeat after three or four days. Also

½ ounce of juice of pineapple leaves may be given twice daily for few days.

Give double the quantities to large animals. Unless the dead worms are expelled from the bowels the animal will die.

When you find the animal will not eat, it must be fed by pouring rice or linseed gruel or barley water down its throat.

After the animal has been purged and the worms passed out, give it a dose of the condition powder (see *Recipes*), every morning for a few weeks, and feed it on warm bran mash for 2 or 3 days.

Accessory Treatment

Keep the animal perfectly clean and warm, free from wet and cold winds. Keep the house and utensils perfectly clean. Remove the dung immediately it is dropped and change the litter every morning; the dung and soiled litter should be burnt. Give the animal plenty of pure drinking-water, fresh, soft, green, grass and bran and oilcake mash. The bran must be steeped in boiling water first. Small calves; kids and lambs should be given warm skimmed milk and rice or linseed *kanji*. Keep the diseased animal apart from the rest.

Preventive

Absolute cleanliness, and sufficient salt and sulphur in the food, and pure drinking-water.

Tuberculosis

Consumption, Tabes, Scrofula, Pining, Grapes, Phthisis in man. In India, the incidence of tuberculosis is far more prevalent than was formerly supposed.

Nature

It is an infectious, incurable disease, common to man and a large number of animals, caused by *bacillus tuberculosis*, and characterized by formation of tubercules in the lungs and other parts of the body. It is usually of a protracted nature.

Susceptibility

Nearly all animals, either naturally or by inoculation. Cattle are very subject to it. Sheep and goats are usually immune. Horses and asses are rarely affected. Is common to birds. Lastly human beings are very susceptible to it.

Infection

The frequency of this disease in human beings and cattle in the same country is almost a proof of their interchangeability from one to the other species.

The infection is by inhalation, ingestion and inoculation. In cattle it is usually by inhalation, and a diseased one infects another in the stable by forcibly expelling the coughed out material containing the germ.

Frequent cause is also by drinking milk from a tubercular patient.

Human beings are similarly infected.

Predisposing causes are heavy milking in cows, breeding too young, in-breeding, debilitating diseases, overcrowding, insanitary surroundings, etc.

Symptoms

Is usually of a chronic nature, and chiefly shows itself in three forms: (1) the lungs; (2) intestinal; (3) mammary.

It may last for months without suspicion.

Lungs Form—Besides the lungs and the pleura the lymphatic glands adjoining it are also involved.

There will be cough, stands upright, pain on pressure over the ribs; later the symptoms are more pronounced and there is fever, etc., and loss of condition even to thinness, and cough more persistent and painful.

The abdominal form which is also termed "Tabes Mesenterica," the intestines, glands, liver, spleen and pancreas, etc., become affected. There is gradual loss of condition in spite of the animal having a good feed, and digestive trouble, *e.g.*, tympany, and irregular bowels, etc.

The mammary form may be from a primary infection from externally of the milk duct but more commonly it is secondary to a generalized case.

At first there is uniform painless swelling of one or more quarters without much disturbance to milk secretion, afterwards gland becomes knotted and the milk turns pale and watery and semi-coagulated. Finally, the udder becomes hard like stone with swelling of the lymphatics near it.

Diagnosis may be confirmed by bacteriological examination or by tuberculine test which is only a diagnostic one in case of a reaction indicated by rise of temperature and swelling at the seat of inoculation.

How to Deal with the Disease

(1) Destroy if possible or dispose off all diagnosed cases particularly if there is emaciation or affection of mammary glands in cows.

(2) In dairy herds if there is any doubt test with tuberculine and destroy or dispose off the reactors.

(3) Imported animals should undergo tuberculine test before purchase or before admission to the dairy herds.

(4) Thoroughly disinfect the standings of affected animals. Pay particular attention to mangers, walls, flooring and bedding or anything contaminated.

(5) Do not use milk from cows with hard udder.

(6) When from loss of condition or chronic wasting an animal is considered suspicious of tuberculosis, boil the milk for half an hour until the tuberculine test shows otherwise.

(7) Milk vessels should be thoroughly cleaned. Steam and boiling water are best for this as medicinal agents taste or spoil the butter and milk.

(8) Flesh of cases in the early stages and if cooked, and any intramuscular glands removed, is fit food; otherwise should not be used.

Treatment

It is not advisable to treat a case of tuberculosis in lower animals, as it is not safe, and the affected animal should be destroyed and buried.

Anthrax

Anthrax also known as Splenic Fever, Malignant Carbuncle, Woolsorter's disease (human), etc., is an acute, highly infectious disease of the cattle, horses, man, etc., caused by the introduction into the system of anthrax micro-organism which remains in the blood circulation and is indicated by high fever, enlarged spleen and collection of blood into the subcutaneous tissues and very sudden death. There are usually two forms–internal and external–of which the internal is generally seen in cattle.

It usually occurs in animals at pasture in marshy, undrained and low soil through the ingestion of food and water containing anthrax spores (egg).

Symptoms

Generally begins by sudden death of one or more animals although in good condition; there is amber coloured condition of mucous membrane of the nostril, eversion of the rectum showing dark coloured membrane, rapid and great decomposition of the carcass after death. There may be difficulty in breathing, convulsion and coming out of blood from nostrils and death occurs either in a few minutes or hours.

Infection

Is carried through the spores in hides, bone-meals, wools, etc., from one country to a distant one.

Treatment

Can only be done at the end of an outbreak which consists of 5 to 10 per cent. solution of carbolic acid into the swelling (external form). The internal form is not amenable to treatment being usually very sudden in its appearance and death.

Prevention

Immunize the healthy animals by protective inoculation by a veterinary surgeon.

Rabies (Hydrophobia in Man)

Causes

Bites from mad dogs, jackals, or other animals.

Symptoms

Cattle, sheep and goats get the *furious* form and show violent symptoms by being very much restless, dash against objects or go for persons, kick, saliva comes out of the mouth, eyes become very red and staring, later become paralytic and die.

Treatment

There is no treatment for this disease; it is best to keep such animal in chains, for 10 days, under observation or to destroy the animal at once, but much may be done to prevent the disease. Experiments are also being made nowadays by which animals bitten, like human beings, are treated with anti-rabic injections in some of the veterinary colleges.

Immediately an animal is bitten, bathe the wound thoroughly and when this has dried, pour a few drops of carbolic or nitric acid into the wound. This will destroy the poison which remains in the saliva of the diseased animal. The saliva of a mad dog becomes poisonous 2 or 3 days before symptoms are shown by it.

Persons and animals bitten or licked on a sore by a mad dog should immediately be sent to the nearest pasteur institute and veterinary college for protective inoculation and treatment. The brain of the mad dog should be sent to the veterinary college for examination.

Recipes

Destroy Maggots

Strong spirits of camphor or oil turpentine poured into the wound, or custard-apple leaves and camphor ground together and put into the wound. Close up the mouth of the wound with lint. Remove the maggots and wash the wound thoroughly every morning and evening with phenyle and warm water before applying the medicine. This should be done until all the maggots are taken out. After that keep the wound clean and dressed with phenyle or carbolic and water.

Horn-oil

Mustard oil, 1 lb.; bees-wax, one ounce; camphor, two ounces; oil of eucalyptus, two ounces.

Hoof-oil

Camphor, 2 ounces; bees-wax, 2 ounces; mustard oil, 8 ounces; turpentine, 2 ounces; and phenyle, 4 ounces.

Purifying Water

Quarter of a teaspoonful of powdered alum and one grain of permanganate of potash in five gallons of water.

How to Administer Medicine

Give the medicine on a small piece of dry bread, or mix up with little honey or treacle (*goorh*), or else make a bamboo tube (*chonga*), or take a long-necked strong bottle, put the liquid medicine in it, make a man hold the animal by the horns, take hold of the creature by the mouth, raise its head up to the level of its back, open the mouth, introduce the *chonga* or, bottle into the mouth and gently pour in a little of the medicine by rotating the bottle from the side of the mouth; as soon as it has swallowed it, more must be given, until the whole is taken. The drench-horn is preferable when at hand.

Care should always be taken, especially in animals suffering from sore-throat, in giving the medicine in small quantities at a time, and if the animal coughs, or attempts to cough, the assistant should at once let go the head so as to allow the animal to depress the head and cough freely and thereby prevent the chance of any of the medicine passing into the windpipe. If the assistant does not let go the head as soon as there is any sign of the animal wishing to cough, some of the medicine may pass into the windpipe and cause death.

N.B.: The tongue must not be pressed on any account and should be allowed to play freely.

Steam-Inhalation

Sprinkle either eucalyptus or turpentine oils 20 to 30 drops in a bucket of steaming hot water and allow the animal to inhale the vapour. Useful for cough, cold and other respiratory troubles.

Gruels

One pound of gram, wheat, rice, barley, or linseed well ground and mixed with two quarts of hot water and properly boiled for half an hour, a dessertspoonful of salt added.

Poultices

Linseed poultice. Grind the linseed into powder, mix some in hot water and place over a fire; stir well until it thickens; place between the folds of a thick piece of cloth, and put it over the affected part.

Bran Poultice

Bran to be so mixed in hot water as to form a soft paste; place on a cloth, pour a little mustard oil over the upper surface, and apply. Should there be any wound, it should be painted with tinct. iodine before, applying the poultice and change it and apply tinct. iodine after washing antiseptically. Useful for reduction of heat and swelling in an inflamed area.

Fumigation

Shed–Burn sulphur (gandhak) in an iron vessel over fire in the empty cow-house with closed doors. Keep the doors closed for four houRs.

Animal–Burn sulphur or tar in an iron vessel over fire in front of the bullock or cow, so that the fumes may be inhaled by the animal. The animal must be placed in an open shed.

In fumigating, care is necessary so that the animal may be able to inhale air as well as the smoke of the sulphur or tar.

The inhaling of the fumes of sulphur and tar alone, without being mixed with sufficient air, would kill an animal.

Fomentation

Boil a lot of *neem* leaves in water or mix up 1 lb. of common salt or Epsom salt in ½ gallon of boiled water, and apply for half an hour soaked in a flannel or blanket cloth, taking care that the part fomented is not chilled; then thoroughly dry the part with dry cloths, and rub in:

Mustard oil	4 ounces
Spirit of turpentine	2 ounces
Camphor	2 ounces

well mixed together; or else rub Elliman's embrocation.

Disinfectants

For the cow-house and shed, phenyle, one part to ten of water. Pure carbolic acid, one part to eight of water. Quick-lime, sprinkled over the floor, and put on the walls. The animal must be taken out of the house while the place is being disinfected.

Vermin Destroyer

Besides the above, the following is very effective: Dry tobacco leaves and catechu soaked in water, and the floor, walls, and wood well rubbed with it. For woodwork nothing is better than kerosene oil nine parts to coal tar one part thoroughly mixed and applied. "Flit " is also very efficacious but costly.

Recipes of Indigenous and Other Drugs

For Diseases Etc.

Medicinal doses must be regulated according to the age, size and condition of the animal. Cattle and sheep at 2 years of age can take full doses, but weak animals (full grown) should be given less and large sized ones more.

The doses in the following recipes are for full grown animals (cattle) unless otherwise stated. Sheep and goats can be given roughly one-sixth of the dose administered to cattle.

Purgatives

	(a)	
(1)	Common salt (namak Lahori)	6 oz. (3 chittacks)
	Epsom salt (jolab-ka-námak)	1 lb. (8 chittacks)
	Ginger (sounth)	1 oz. (½ chittack)
	Treacle (goorh)	8 oz. (4 chittacks)

To be well mixed up in a quart of hot water (1½ seers) and given warm.

This is for a full grown cow, bullock or buffalo; give half the quantity to a small full grown animal and one-sixth to a full grown sheep.

(b)	
(2) Linseed oil (alsi-ka-tel)	10 oz. (5 chittacks)
Sweet oil (mitha-tel)	10 oz. (5 chittacks)
Croton oil (jamalgotta-ka-tel)	30 mus. (30 katras)

Mix together and give to a full grown animal as a purgative–one-sixth for sheep.

Mild Purgatives

(a)	
(3) Common salt (námak Lahori)	4 oz. (2 chittacks)
Powdered sulphur (gandhak)	3 oz. (1½ chittacks)
Powdered ginger (sounth)	4 dr. (¼ chittack)
Treacle (goorh)	3 oz. (1½ chittacks)

To be well mixed up in a quart of hot water (¼ seer) and given warm.

(b)	
(4) Castor oil (rerhi-ka-tel)	10 oz. (5 chittacks)
Linseed oil (alsi-ka-tel)	6 oz. (3 chittacks)

Mix well and give as mild purgative for cattle. One-sixth for sheep and calves.

For Fever

(a)	
(5) Common salt (námak Lahori)	10 oz. (2½ tolas)
Nitre (shora)	4 dr. (1¼ tolas)
Powdered chiretta	1 oz. (2½ tolas)
Treacle (goorh)	4 oz. (2 chittacks)

To be given in a pint of water.

(b)

(6)	Camphor (kafur)	2 dr. (6 two-anna bits)
	Nitre (shora)	3 dr. (1 tola)
	Arrack (shurab)	2 oz. (1 chittack)

Dissolve the camphor in spirit, then add nitre and arrack and give in a pint of water.

(c)

(7)	Epsom salt	6 oz. (3 chittacks)
	Ammon. chlor. (nashadar)	3 dr. (1 tola)
	Nitre (shora)	3 dr. (1 tola)

To be given in 2 pints of water.

Astringent Powder for Obstinate Diarrhoea in Cattle

(8)	Powdered chalk (khariamati)	1 oz. (½ chittack)
	Catechu (katha)	½ oz. (¼ chittack)
	Ginger (sounth)	½ oz. (¼ chittack)
	Opium (aphim)	1 dr. (3 two-anna bits)
	Arrack (shurab)	2 oz. (1 chittack)

Mix thoroughly and give in a pint of rice gruel, twice daily until diarrhoea stops.

Astringent Mixture

(9)	Acid sulphuric dil.	1 oz. (1 chittack)
	Infusion chiretta (chereita-ka-pani)	1 pint (10 chittacks)

Mix and give in rice gruel, twice daily until diarrhoea stops.

For Diarrhoea due to Bad Liver

When the dung becomes blackish or clay coloured and there is very offensive smell.

(10) Acid nitro muriatic dil	1 dr. (60 drops or katras).
Infusion chiretta (chereita-ka-pani)	1 pint (10 chittacks).

Mix thoroughly and give with or without food, twice daily.

For Diarrhoea and Dysentery in Calves

(11) Castor oil (rerhi-ka-tel)	1 oz. (½ chittack).
Turpentine oil (tarpin-ka-tel)	30 mns. (30 katras).
Mucilage acacia (babul-ka-gaundh) little.	
Camphor water (kafur-ka-pani)	2 oz. (1 chittack).

Mix the first two thoroughly with mucilage and then add water and give according to necessity.

When the diarrhoea commences, give lime water one ounce with milk, twice daily.

For Hoven (Tympany)

(12) Oil, turpentine (tarpin-ka-tel)	1 oz. (½ chittack).
Asafoetida powder (hing)	4 dr. (¼ chittack).
Oil, linseed (alsi-ka-tel)	1 pint (10 chittacks).

Dissolve the asafoetida with turpentine and then add linseed oil and mix up thoroughly and give at once and repeat if necessary after 3 or 4 hours.

For Impaction of the Stomach

(13) Powdered nux vom. (kuchla)	1 dr. (3 two-anna bits).
Epsom salt (jolab-ka-námak)	8 oz. (4 chittacks).
Common salt (namak Lahori)	4 oz. (2 chittacks).
Powdered ginger (sounth)	1 oz. (1½ tolas).
Arrack (shurab)	2 oz. (1 chittack).
Water (lukewarm)	1½ pints (about 1 seer).

Mix up the above thoroughly in water and give when warm, followed by one pint of linseed oil if necessary.

Cleansing Draught for Retention of After-Birth

(14) Ext. ergot. liq.	1 dr. (60 minims).
Common salt (námak Lahori)	6 oz. (3 chittacks).
Arrack (shurab)	4 oz. (2 chittacks).
Water	1 pint (10 chittacks).

Mix up the above and give internally.

Stimulants

(15) Powdered ginger (sounth)	1 oz. (½ chittack).
Powdered black pepper (kala mirich)	½ oz. (¼ chittack).
Arrack (shurab)	4 oz. (2 chittacks).

Mix up thoroughly and give in a quart of water and repeat whenever necessary.

Rum, brandy, or arrack in 2 to 4 ounces may also be given with a pint (10 chittacks) of water or rice gruel, and repeated if necessary.

Condition Powder or Tonic Powder

(a)	
(16) Black salt	1 seer.
Sulphur	½ seer.
Dried ginger	½ seer.
Chiretta (powdered)	½ seer.
Camphor	½ seer.
Ajwain (Bishop seed)	½ seer.
Mustard seed	½ seer.
Methee	½ seer.
Turmeric	½ seer.

All to be well powdered and mixed together. From ½ to 1 ounce to be given to each animal every morning and evening. Half the quantity for goats, sheep, and calves. Continue for a fortnight.

(b)

(17) Powdered nux vom.	½ to 1 dr.
Powdered gentian	2 to 4 dr.
Powdered ginger	2 to 4 dr.
Powdered columba	2 to 4 dr.
Soda bicarb.	2 to 4 dr.
Ammon. chlor.	2 to 4 dr.

Mix up the above and give with food twice daily. Very good tonic.

Anodyne (To relieve pain)

(a)

(18) Leaves of Indian hemp (bhang)	3 dr. (1 tola).
Asafoetida (hing)	3 dr. (1 tola).

Mix up thoroughly the leaves with little water and make it into a paste and then add asafoetida and afterwards add a pint of water or gruel and give as drench.

(b)

(19) Opium (aphim)	3 dr. (1 tola).
Asafoetida (hing)	3 dr. (1 tola).
Ginger (sounth)	4 dr. (2 chittacks).
Black pepper (kala mirich)	1 dr. (1 tola).

All to be powdered and mixed in a pint of water or gruel and given as a drench.

(c)

(20) Chloral hydras	1 oz.
Mucilage acacia (babul-ka-gaundh)	½ oz.
Water or gruel	2 pints.

Mix up thoroughly the first and the second ingredients with little water and then gradually add more water up to 2 pints and give as drench. Repeat if necessary.

Vermifuge (For removal of intestinal worms)

(a)

(21) Oil turpentine (tarpin-ka-tel)	2 oz. (1 chittack).
Linseed oil (alsi-ka-tel)	1 pint (10 chittacks).

Give as a drench after starving the animal for 8 to 12 hours.

(b)

(22) Common salt (námak Lahori)	1 oz. (1 chittack).
Powdered sulphate of iron (hirakash)	½ oz. (¼ chittack).
Powdered sulphur (gandhak)	1 oz. (½ chittack).

Mix up well and give twice daily in a quart of water and follow with a purgative.

For Cough and Cold

(23) Powdered camphor (kafur)	1 dr. (3 two-anna bits).
Powdered ginger (sounth)	1 oz. (½ chittack).
Ammon. chlor. (nashadar)	2 dr. (1/8 chittack).
or	
Potash. chlor.	2 dr. (1/8 chittack).

Powder well and mix up thoroughly with treacle and place it over the tongue twice daily.

For External use

Eye Lotion

(24) Boracic acid	5 gr.
Alum (phitkiri)	2 gr.
Distilled water	1 oz.

Mix up thoroughly and drop into the affected eyes 3 or 4 times a day. Put a bandage over the eye.

For Burns and Scalds

Apply immediately one of the following over the parts.

(25) 1. Methylated spirit or whisky, brandy or absolute alcohol.
2. Treacle.
3. Potato made into a paste.
4. Carron oil (stir thoroughly lime water and coconut oil equal quantity).
5. Saturated sol. of tannic acid.

N.B.: Do not apply any water over the affected parts.

Anodyne Applications (For Swelling and Pain)

(a)

Belladonna Liniments

(26) Camphor	1 part.
Liq. ext. belladonna	10 parts.
Alcohol	7 parts.
Distilled water	2 parts.

All properly mixed together, to be applied with a soft brush over the affected parts.

(b)

Camphor Liniments

(27) Camphor	1 part.
Oil olive	4 parts.

Dissolve the camphor in spirit and then add the oil; mix up and apply.

(c)

(28) Turpentine oil	1 part.
Camphor	½ part.
Mustard oil	10 parts.

First heat the /mustard oil and then add camphor and turpentine. Stir it well and rub over the affected part while warm with friction.

Mange Dressing

(29) Powdered sulphur (gandhak)	4 oz. (2 chittacks).
Kerosene oil	4 oz. (2 chittacks).
Rape oil (karua tel)	1 pint (10 chittacks).

Mix and rub a portion of the affected part twice daily with friction.

Mouth Gargle or Wash

(30) Alum (phitkiri)	4 dr. (1½ tolas).
Borax (shohaga)	4 dr. (1½ tolas).
Water	1 pint (10 chittacks).

Dissolve and use as a mouth wash and healing lotion for wounds inside the mouth.

Dusting Powder for Wounds

(31) Iodoform	1 part.
Zinc oxide	2 parts.
Boric acid	3 parts.
Starch	4 parts.

Mix up the above ingredients together thoroughly and dust over the wounds.

Breeder's Table

Time of Service		*Mares 340 days*		*Cows 283 days*		*Ewes 150 days*		*Sows 112 days*		*Bitches 63 days*	
Jan	1	Dec	6	Oct	10	May	30	April	22	March	4
Jan	8	Dec	13	Oct	17	June	6	April	29	March	11
Jan	15	Dec	20	Oct	24	June	13	May	6	March	18
Jan	22	Dec	27	Oct	31	June	20	May	13	March	25
Jan	29	Jan	3	Nov	7	June	27	May	20	April	1
Feb	5	Jan	10	Nov	14	July	4	May	27	April	8
Feb	12	Jan	17	Nov	21	July	11	June	3	April	15
Feb	19	Jan	24	Nov	28	July	18	June	10	April	22
Feb	26	Jan	31	Dec	5	July	25	June	17	April	29
March	5	Feb	7	Dec	12	Aug	1	June	24	May	6
March	12	Feb	14	Dec	19	Aug	8	July	1	May	13
March	19	Feb	21	Dec	26	Aug	15	July	8	May	20
March	26	Feb	28	Jan	2	Aug	22	July	15	May	27
April	2	March	7	Jan	9	Aug	29	July	22	June	3
April	9	March	14	Jan	16	Sep	5	July	29	June	10
April	16	March	21	Jan	23	Sep	12	Aug	5	June	17
April	23	March	28	Jan	30	Sep	19	Aug	12	June	24
April	30	April	4	Feb	6	Sep	26	Aug	19	July	1
May	7	April	11	Feb	13	Oct	3	Aug	26	July	8
May	14	April	18	Feb	20	Oct	10	Sep	2	July	15
May	21	April	25	Feb	27	Oct	17	Sep	9	July	22

contd...

Contd...

Time of Service	Mares 340 days	Cows 283 days	Ewes 150 days	Sows 112 days	Bitches 63 days
May 28	May 2	March 6	Oct 24	Sep 16	July 29
June 4	May 9	March 13	Oct 31	Sep 23	Aug 5
June 11	May 16	March 20	Nov 7	Sep 30	Aug 12
June 18	May 23	March 27	Nov 14	Oct 7	Aug 19
June 25	May 30	April 3	Nov 21	Oct 14	Aug 26
July 2	June 6	April 10	Nov 28	Oct 21	Sep 2
July 9	June 13	April 17	Dec 5	Oct 28	Sep 9
July 16	June 20	April 24	Dec 12	Nov 4	Sep 16
July 23	June 27	May 1	Dec 19	Nov 11	Sep 23
July 30	July 4	May 8	Dec 26	Nov 18	Sep 30
Aug 6	July 11	May 15	Jan 2	Nov 25	Oct 7
Aug 13	July 18	May 22	Jan 9	Dec 2	Oct 14
Aug 20	July 25	May 29	Jan 16	Dec 9	Oct 21
Aug 27	Aug 1	June 5	Jan 23	Dec 16	Oct 28
Sep 3	Aug 8	June 12	Jan 30	Dec 23	Nov 4
Sep 10	Aug 15	June 19	Feb 6	Dec 30	Nov 11
Sep 17	Aug 22	June 26	Feb 13	Jan 6	Nov 18
Sep 24	Aug 29	July 3	Feb 20	Jan 13	Nov 25
Oct 1	Sep 5	July 10	Feb 27	Jan 20	Dec 2
Oct 8	Sep 12	July 17	March 6	Jan 27	Dec 9
Oct 15	Sep 19	July 24	March 13	Feb 3	Dec 16
Oct 22	Sep 26	July 31	March 20	Feb 10	Dec 23
Oct 29	Oct 3	Aug 7	March 27	Feb 17	Dec 30
Nov 5	Oct 10	Aug 14	April 3	Feb 24	Jan 6
Nov 12	Oct 17	Aug 21	April 10	March 3	Jan 13
Nov 19	Oct 24	Aug 28	April 17	March 10	Jan 20
Nov 26	Oct 31	Sep 4	April 24	March 17	Jan 27
Dec 3	Nov 7	Sep 11	May 1	March 24	Feb 3
Dec 10	Nov 14	Sep 18	May 8	March 31	Feb 10
Dec 17	Nov 21	Sep 25	May 15	April 7	Feb 17
Dec 24	Nov 28	Oct 2	May 22	April 14	Feb 24
Dec 31	Dec 5	Oct 9	May 29	April 21	March 3

Weights and Measures

Measures of Capacity

1 Minim (*m*)	=	1 Drop (Katra)
60 Minims (*m*)	=	1 Drachm (3)–1/16 Chittack
1 Drachm (fluid)	=	1/16 Chittack–one teaspoonful
2 Drachms (fluid)	=	1/8 Chittack
4 Drachms (fluid)	=	¼ Chittack–one tablespoonful
8 Drachms (fluid)	=	1 Ounce (3)–½ Chittack
2 Ounces	=	1 Chittack
20 Ounces	=	1 Pint–10 Chittacks
4 Gills	=	1 Pint–10 Chittacks
2 Pints	=	1 Quart–1¼ Seers–20 Chittacks
2 Quarts	=	1 Bottle–2½ Seers
4 Quarts	=	1 Gallon–5 Seers
2 Gallons	=	1 Peck–10 Seers
4 Pecks	=	1 Bushel–1 Maund
2 Bushels	=	1 Strike–2 Maunds
3 Bushels	=	1 Sack–3 Maunds
8 Bushels	=	1 Quarter–8 Maunds
12 Sacks	=	1 Chaldron–36 Maunds
5 Quarters	=	1 Wey or Load–40 Maunds
10 Quarters	=	1 Last–80 Maunds

Avoirupois Weight

16 Drams	=	1 Ounce (oz.)–(437½ grains)– ½ Chittack-2½ Tolas.
16 Ounces	=	1 Pound (lb.)–½ Seer.
14 Pounds	=	1 Stone–7 SeeRs.
28 Pounds	=	1 Quarter–14 SeeRs.
112 Pounds	=	1 Hundredweight (cwt.)–1 Maund, 16 Seers (4 quarters).
20 Hundredweights	=	1 Ton-28 Maunds.
A Pound Avoir.	=	7,000 Grains Troy.

Square and Land Measure

144 Inches	=	1 Square Foot
9 Feet	=	I Square Yard
30¼ Yards	=	1 Square Rod, Pole or Perch
16 Poles	=	1 Chain
40 Poles	=	1 Rood
4 Roods	=	1 Acre (4.840 yards)
640 Acres	=	1 Square Mile (1,760 yards)

Bengal Square or Land Measure

5 Haths Long × 4 Broad	=	1 Chittack
1 Chittack	=	45 sq. ft. or 5 sq. yds.
16 Chittacks	=	1 Cottah = 720 sq. ft. or 80 sq. yds.
20 Cottahs	=	1 Bigha = 14,400 sq. ft. or 1,600 sq. yds.
3 Bighas	=	1 Acre.

Bazaar Weight

4 Sicki	=	1 Tola–1 rupee–3 drams.
5 Sicki	=	1 Kancha–1¼ rupee weight.
4 Kanchas	=	1 Chittack–5 rupees weight.
4 Chittacks	=	1 Powah–20 rupees weight.
4 Powahs	=	1 Seer–80 rupees weight.
5 Seers	=	1 Pussaree–10 lb. or 10 lb. 10 oz.
8 Pussarees	=	1 Maund–80 or 82½ lb.
Four bundles of straw or hay make one Gonda.		
20 Gondas	=	1 Pon.
16 Pons	=	1 Kahon.

Apothecaries' Weight

(Measures of Weight)

20 Grains	=	1 Scrouple (1 scr.) or 2 two-anna bits.
3 Scrouples	=	1 Drachm (1 dr.)
8 Drachms	=	1 Ounce Troy.

Indian Names of Some Cattle Diseases

Rinderpest or Cattle Plague	Gooti-Mata-Mohamari, Boshonto.
Malignant Sore-Throat	Gulaphula-Galsuja.
Anthrax	Tarka-Paschima-Goli.
Black-quarter	Badhla-Badarkhor-Sujwa
Foot-and-Mouth	Khuria-Khurpacha-Aensho
Red-Water	Roktomutra-Lalpishab
Cow-pox	Mata-Boshonto-Gooti
Tuberculosis	Khansi-Kashi-Jokkha-Khai Kâsh
Inflammation of the Udder	Thunkah-Thanphula, Palanphula
Cough	Khânshi
Hopven (Tympanitis)	Pate-phola
Diarrhoea and Scours	Chærta-Pate-nabano
Epilepsy	Mirgi
Grains-Sick	Simla

Indigenous Drugs with their Vernacular Names and Purposes

Name of Medicines	*Vernacular Names*		*Purpose for which Used*	*Dose*
	Hindustani	*Bengali*		
Alum	Phitkiri	Phatkiri	Astringent, checks milk secretion	1-2 dr.
Aloes	Musabbar	Masabbar	Tonic and purgative	4-6 dr.
Aniseed	Sonf	Mauri	Aromatic for digestive trouble	1-2 oz.
Arrack (country liquor)	Shurab	Madh	Stimulant	4-8 oz.
Asafoetida	Hing	Hing	Flatulence, gripes and worms	2-4 oz.
Black pepper	Kala mirich	Gol-marich	Stimulant and digestive	2-4 oz.
Black salt	Kala námak	Kalo-nun	Digestive and tonic	2-4 oz.
Borax	Shohaga	Sohaga	Astringent and antiseptic for mouth wash	2-4 oz.
Castor oil	Rerhi-ka-tel	Rehrir-tel	Laxative	1-2 oz. (calf)

contd...

Contd...

Name of Medicines	Vernacular Names		Purpose for which Used	Dose
	Hindustani	Bengali		
Camphor	Kafur	Karpur	Stimulant (cough and cold) gripes	½-2 pints (cows)
Caradamom	Elaichee	Elach	Aromatic and digestive	2-4 oz.
Catechu	Katha	Khair	Astringent for diarrhoea	2-4 oz.
Chalk	Khariamati	Khari	Astringent for diarrhoea	2-4 oz.
Charcoal	Koila	Kath-koila	Absorbent for flatulence	1-2 oz.
Chireta powder	Chereita	Chirata	Bitter tonic	2-4 oz.
Common salt	Námak	Laban	Purgative and digestive	1-2 lb.
Croton oil	Jamalgotta-ka-tel	Jaipal	Drastic purgative	30-40 mns.
Copper sulph.	Tootia	Tute	Vermituge and caustic	1-2 dr.
Ginger	Sounth	Suth	Aromatic and corrective	4-8 dr.
Gum acacia or Gum arabic	Gaundh	Bablar-atha	Astringent and soothing for stomach	4-8 dr.
Indian hemp (leaves) (Cannabis indica)	Bhang	Sidddhi	Reduces pain and induces sleep	1-2 dr.
— Do — (extract)	Charas	Charas	— Do —	
Indra jab		Indra jab	Soothing to stomach and intestines	1-2 oz.
Ishapgul seed	Ishapgul	Ishapgul	Cooling to the bowels, for dysentery	1-2 oz.
Kerosene oil	Mitti-ka-tel	Kerasin tel	Parasiticide for skin disease	(externally)

contd...

Contd...

Name of Medicines	*Vernacular Names*		*Purpose for which Used*	*Dose*
	Hindustani	*Bengali*		
Lime water	Chuna-ka-pani	Chuner-jal	Antacid for dyspepsia and diarrhoea in calves	2-4 oz.
Linseed	Alsi	Tishi	Soothing to stomach and urinary tracts	Q.S.
Linseed oil	Alsi-ka-tel	Tishir-tel	Laxative and soothing	1-2 pints.
Nux vomica	Kuchla	Kunchla	Stimulant, bitter and nerve tonic	1-2 dr.
Opium	Aphim	Aphing	Astringent and anodine	1-3 dr
Omum (Bishop seed)	Ajowan	Jowain	Stimulant and carminative	1-2 dr.
Sulphur	Gandhak	Gandhak	Alterative and laxative	3-4 dr.
Sulphate of iron (ferri sulph.)	Hirakash	Heerakash	Tonic (blood) anthelmintic	1-2 dr.
Sal-ammoniac (ammon. chlor.)	Nashadar	Nishedal	Cooling for fever and liver trouble	2-4 dr.
Tobacco leaves	Tamaku-ka-patti	Tamak-pata	Parasiticide for skin disease and removal of ticks and lice	(externally)
Turpentine oil	Tarpin-ka-tel	Tarpin-tel	For worms (intestinal) and for hoven. Externally anodyne	1-2 oz.
Treacle (jagri)	Sheera	Goorh	Laxative	1-2 lb.
Vasaka	Arusha	Basak or Bakash	Expectorant for cough and cold	1-2 oz. 2-4 oz. (juice) (leaves)

Index

A

Advantages of keeping cows, 3-5
Anthrax, 212
Artifical milk of calves and pigs, 205
Attendants, 82-83

B

Barren cows, 124-127
Bhainsha *ghee*, 174
Bhoosa (chaff), 103, 114, 157, 181, 182, 211
Bran, 211
Braxy in sheep, 212
Breeding, 86, 170, 177, 191-197, 202
Breeds of cattle, 6
  Amrit Mahal Bullocks, 35
  Awankari breed, 37
  Ayrshire cow, Dewdrop, 46, 94, 189
  Bengali, 37-42, 38
  Bhagalpore cattle, 43
  Bihar cattle, 42-43
  Brahmami bull, 27
  breed to get, 50
  cross Hansi country, 24
  cross-breed English cows, 45
  Darjeeling cattle, 43-45
  Dhanni cattle, 34-37
  English and Australian cattle, 45
  gir (Kathiawar), 26-31, 33
  Hansi, 19, 20, 22, 23
  Hansi or Hissar, 12
  Hilstein cow, 49
  Hissar breed, 16, 17, 18
  jersey cow, 48
  Kangayam, 34
  kankreji cattle, 31
  Krishna valley cattle, 34
  montgomery bull (Amritsari), 7, 8, 9-11, 113, 137, 170
  Mooltan and Amritsar cows, 31-33
  Mysore bullocks, 34
  Mysore-Nadu bull, 36
  Nagpuri, 16-25
  Nellore or Ongole, 26
  Ongole, 28-30
  Patna cattle, 45-50
  price of a pair of good bullocks, 26
  pure Siri cow, 44
  Shahabad, 39, 40, 41

short-thorn dairy cow, 47
sind, 12-16
trotting bullocks, 16
young Hansi bull, 21

Bullocks, 98-99
Bulls, 93-97
Butter, 146, 166
Buying cows, 51-54

C

Calves, 111-116
Castrating calves, 118-119
Cattle show, 182
Cattle-breeding in India, 185-189
Cattle-dung, 159
Chamar, 250
Chapped teats, 138
Chonga, 282
Cotton-seed, 102
Country-bred cow, 203
Cows milk, 174
Cream, 143, 146, 147, 148
Cross-breds, 170
Curd, cheese and tyer, 153, 154

D

Dairy, 170
farming, 168-172, 189, 191

Dairyman, 175
Diseases, 200
abscess, 252
apoplexy, 244-245
calving, 226
causes of ropy milk, 231-232
choking, 238-240
colic or gripes (pain in the abdomen), 246-247
cure for mastitis, 231-232
epilepsy, 243-244
fardel-bound, 236-238
flooding, 226-227
grain sick, 235-236
hernia, 250
hoven, 233-235
hydatids (bladder-worms), 248-249
indigestion and diarrhea, 242-243
inflammation of the bowels (enteritis), 249-252
inflammation of the brain, 245-246
inflammation of the womb (metritis), 227-228
jaundice, 250
mammitis or swollen udder, 229-231
paralysis, 233
parasitic warbles, 247-248
poisoning, 250
red-water, 240-242
rheumatism, 232
slipping down of the womb, 228-229
treatment for lumpy milk, 231

Diseases of cattle, goats and sheep, 211
carcasses, 214
contagious diseases, 214
foot-and-mouth disease, 212
hides of cattle, 215
mange in cattle, 215
phenyle, 214
poles of carts and harness, or sladdlery, 215
rinderpest, 214
rules should be strictly adhered, 212
scab in sheep, 215

Dry-cow farming, 177
Duhhee, 154
Dustoori or bribes, 175
Dustoori, 52, 53

E

Earthen (*mutti*) *handi*, 154
Elliman's embrocation, 232, 283
English method of hand feeding, 112
Exercise, 85
Express dairy-farm, 176

F

Farm journal, 54
Fatal diseases, 253, 270, 272
  anthrax, 278-279
  black-quarter (called black-leg or quarter-ill), 265-267
  bronchitis from worms, 264-265
  bronchitis, 262-263
  calf scours, 273-274
  cow-pox (variola), 269-270
  dysentery, 267-268
  foot and mouth disease, 257-261
  how to deal with the disease, 278
  malignant sore-throat (haemorrhagic septicaemia), 261-262
  rabies (hydrophobia in man), 279-280
  rinderpast (cattle–plague), 253
  scours in calves, 274
  slinking or abortion, 268-269
  symptoms: *abdominal form*, 277
  symptoms: *lungs form*, 277
  symptoms: *mammary form*, 277-278
  tuberculosis, 276-278
  white scours in calves, 272-273
  worms in the intestines, 274-276
Flies, 155
Food, 65-73
Frost, J.N., 231
Full-handed milking, 55
Fumigating, 283

G

Ghee, 151, 160
Ginger and *huldi*, 108
Gir breeds, 134
Government Military Dairies in India, 189, 191
Government Military or Agricultural Dairies, 168
Gowah ghee, 174
Gowallas, 122, 175, 176, 203, 180
Grass-lands, 170
Graze during at the rains, 212
Grazing fields, 160-162
Grooming, 84
Guernseys, 188
Gurh (molasses), 108
Gurh-jaggery, 113

H

Haemorrhagic, 212
Handis, 154
Hay, 211
Heifers, 114
Holstein, 188
House and utensils, 75-80
Howman, H.A., 174
Huldi (turmeric), 108, 118

I

Imperial Government, 191
Improvement of cattle in Bengal, 206
Indian cow as a Dairy Animal, 189-190
Indian names at different ages, 128, 132
Indian names of cattle diseases, 298

J

Jhule, 157

K

Kallaie, 102
Keatinge, G.F., 183
Keventer's Dairy-farms, 176
Khansamaship's patronage, 53
Kutheela, 123

L

Libitum, 113
Lice, 155

M

Management of cows when calving, 106-109
Milk, 135, 146, 147, 160, 166, 170
Milking qualities, 58
Mofussil, 134

N

Neem leaves, 232, 283

O

Oil cake, 102, 113

P

Palani, 52
Pinjarapols, 180
Points in a good cow, 57-62
Poshani, 52
Postures, 211
Prices of
 bullocks, 134
 bulls, 134
 calves, 134
 cows, 133-134
Protection, 85
Pure breeds, 170
Pure-bred cows, 134

R

Rearing farms, 176, 177
Rearing of calves in India, 197
Recipes, 281
Regularity in feedings, 113
Religious belief, 190
Rinderpest, 212
Ryots, 133, 160

S

Seasons of the year, 157
Septicaemia, 212
Servant's tricks, 53
Shorthorn bulls, 188
Smith, W.M., 89
Stock of hay, 157
Straw, 211
Sweet oil, 108

T

Taking the bull, 120-122
Taper, 55
Teeth at different ages, 129, 130
Ticks, 155

V

Vaseline, 108
Vegetable ghee, 174
Veterinary surgeon, 54

W

Washing, 84
Wicked practice of *phooka*, 122

Z

Zamindar, 91, 160, 189